Heinemann is an imprint of Pearson Education Limited, a company incorporated in England and Wales, having its registered office at Edinburgh Gate, Harlow, Essex, CM20 2JE. Registered company number: 872828

www.heinemann.co.uk

Heinemann is a registered trademark of Pearson Education Limited

Text © Susan Cressy 2008

First published 2008

12 11 10 09 08
10 9 8 7 6 5 4 3 2 1

British Library Cataloguing in Publication Data is available from the British Library on request.

ISBN 978 0 435449 12 4

Typeset and illustrated by Saxon Graphics Ltd, Derby
Original illustrations © Pearson Education Limited 2008
Cover photo/illustration © Corbis/Punchstock RF
Printed in China

Illustrated Beauty Therapy Dictionary

Susan Cressy

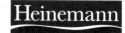

Contents

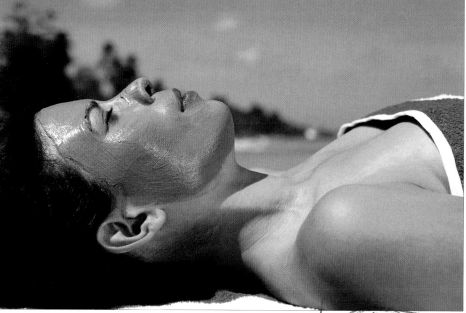

Acknowledgements

The authors and publisher would like to thank the following individuals and organisations for permission to reproduce copyright material.

I would like to thank the following people:

As always my family for their constant support and encouragement

My past and present students for giving me the reason to continue writing

Clare Loftus whose dedication to 'Skills for Life', inspired the idea for a beauty therapy dictionary and Helen, Pat, Kathleen, Leslie, Bev and Alex for making our lessons so entertaining!

BABOR UK and Ireland for providing photographic illustrations

Martin Hamilton, Trafford College for his photographic illustration

Jilly Hunt, Julie Bennett, Juliet Mozley, Olwen Turchetta, from Heinemann and Melanie Birdsall for their help and assistance in publishing this dictionary

Photos
Alamy/Arclight: page 69
ALAN OLIVER/Alamy: page 59
Babor UK and Ireland: pages 161, 175
Corbis: pages iii, 9, 23, 26, 42, 54, 57, 61, 111
f1 online/Alamy: pages 1, 16, 155
Getty Images/Digital Vision: page 156
Getty Images/PhotoDisc: pages 7, 10, 17, 28, 33, 100, 106, 109, 119, 125, 125, 151, 153,166, 186
iStockphoto/Allison Marles: page 149
JOHN RADCLIFFE HOSPITAL/SCIENCE PHOTO LIBRARY: page 88
Martin Hamilton: page 4
Nice Pak International Limited: page 63
Pearson Education ltd./Gareth Bowden: pages 36, 44, 49, 67, 83, 132, 139, 145
Real Health and Beauty by Warren Diggles/ Alamy: page 65
SCIENCE PHOTO LIBRARY/DR P. MARAZZI: pages 37, 39, 81, 90
SCIENCE PHOTO LIBRARY/SCOTT CAMAZINE: page 129
Stephen Frink Collection/Alamy: page 146

Introduction

In the ever-changing world of beauty therapy, you may be faced with many new words and phrases that are both technical and sometimes difficult to pronounce. These words need to be learned as they are part of the essential knowledge required to reinforce the practical skills in beauty, holistic or spa therapy. As well as being able to pronounce the words correctly in order to sound professional and authoritative, it is also important to be able to spell them correctly for written assessment.

This dictionary provides a comprehensive list of all the terms used in beauty therapy and for all awarding bodies. Although it is intended primarily for students of beauty therapy, it will also be useful for anyone embarking on a course in holistic therapy, spa therapy, reflexology, body massage, aromatherapy, Indian head massage, nail treatments or makeup.

Each entry contains a simple definition and, in some cases, a more detailed explanation or description. This will help you to understand the technical information and to check difficult spellings, while also providing a quick source of reference and a valuable resource for revision.

A feature of the dictionary is that it has been written in clear and concise English without the use of unnecessary technical jargon. It also has a pronunciation guide for each word, making the more difficult words easier to say. Words within an entry that are highlighted in bold italic type are also defined in the dictionary.

The dictionary defines many terms in anatomy and physiology, health and safety practice, all the practical skills for beauty, spa and holistic therapies from level 1 to level 3, the business terminology and the professional vocabulary used by all awarding bodies.

The appendix contains full colour diagrams and charts to provide easy access to some of the essential anatomy and physiology information relating to each skill area.

Guide to using this book

The term is given in bold.

The pronunciation is in italics.

Some entries refer to the appendix.

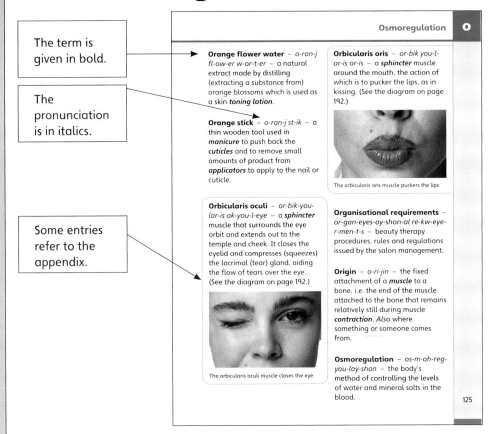

Osmoregulation

o

Orange flower water – *o-ran-j fl-ow-er w-or-t-er* – a natural extract made by distilling (extracting a substance from) orange blossoms which is used as a skin *toning lotion*.

Orange stick – *o-ran-j st-ik* – a thin wooden tool used in *manicure* to push back the *cuticles* and to remove small amounts of product from *applicators* to apply to the nail or cuticle.

Orbicularis oculi – *or-bik-you-lar-is ok-you-l-eye* – a *sphincter* muscle that surrounds the eye orbit and extends out to the temple and cheek. It closes the eyelid and compresses (squeezes) the lacrimal (tear) gland, aiding the flow of tears over the eye. (See the diagram on page 192.)

The orbicularis oculi muscle closes the eye

Orbicularis oris – *or-bik you-l-ar-is or-is* – a *sphincter* muscle around the mouth, the action of which is to pucker the lips, as in kissing. (See the diagram on page 192.)

The orbicularis oris muscle puckers the lips

Organisational requirements – *or-gan-eyes-ay-shon-al re-kw-eye-r-men-t-s* – beauty therapy procedures, rules and regulations issued by the salon management.

Origin – *o-ri-jin* – the fixed attachment of a *muscle* to a bone, i.e. the end of the muscle attached to the bone that remains relatively still during muscle *contraction*. *Also* where something or someone comes from.

Osmoregulation – *os-m-oh-reg-you-lay-shon* – the body's method of controlling the levels of water and mineral salts in the blood.

125

Abdomen – *ab-do-men* – the largest cavity in the body, lying between the chest and the hips. It contains the stomach, intestines, liver, spleen, **pancreas**, kidneys, bladder and **reproductive** organs.

Abduction – *ab-duk-shon* – movement of the limbs away from the **midline** of the body.

Abrasion – *ab-ray-shon* – the act of rubbing or wearing away by friction. Abrasion is used in exfoliation. It is carried out either manually, using products to exfoliate dead skin cells, or using an electrical **treatment** called **microdermabrasion**. Also refers to a scrape on the skin, caused by injury or irritation.

Abscess – *ab-sess* – a localised (in one place) collection of pus in the body caused by **infection**, often accompanied by swelling and **inflammation**.

Absorption – *ab-s-or-p-shon* – the uptake of substances by a body tissue, through a process such as **osmosis** or **diffusion**. For example, the movement of the products of **digestion** through the walls of the small intestine into the blood.

ACAS (Advisory, Conciliation and Arbitration Service) – *ay-k-ass* – an impartial organisation that helps to resolve disputes or disagreements at work *(continued)*

Abrasives – *ab-ray-sivs* – small solid particles used as part of cosmetic products to remove or break up the surface of the skin. They are especially useful for removing hard skin during a **pedicure** or dry skin on the body or face, to improve texture.

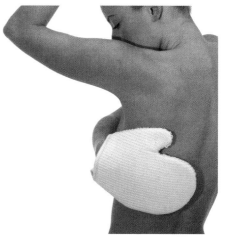

A body scrub

without the need to go to court or a tribunal.

Accessory – *ak-sess-or-ree* – a removable part that makes something complete – for example, a glass **electrode**, a brush or another **applicator** used for a specialised electrical **treatment**. Also an additional item that **enhances** an outfit, e.g. a handbag or earrings.

Accounts – *ak-ow-n-ts* – a summary of the financial transactions of a business, with details of the turnover and profit in a given period. Usually prepared by an accountant for tax purposes.

Acetone – *a-set-oh-n* – a colourless, volatile (evaporates rapidly), water-soluble (dissolves in water), **flammable** liquid. Used as a **solvent** in nail enamel remover and to remove false nails from the natural nail plate.

Acid mantle – *a-sid man-tul* – a thin, oily layer on the surface of the skin that forms part of the body's defence system. It is made up of **sebum** and sweat and has a natural **acidity**, with a **pH** value of 4–5.5. This helps prevent **bacterial** growth on the skin and hair. Many of the harmful substances that might enter the skin, such as chemicals from the atmosphere and harmful bacteria, are **alkaline**. The acid mantle neutralises these chemicals and bacteria. Maintaining the skin's pH at the proper level is vital to protecting ourselves from harmful bacteria that can lead to **acne**, **infection** or **irritation**.

Acidity – *a-sid-it-ee* – the state of being acid (sour). Also the measurement of how acid a substance is. Acidity is measured on the **pH** scale and acids have pH values below 7.

Acne vulgaris – *ak-nee vul-gar-ris* – the most common type of acne. It is an **inflammation** of the **sebaceous glands**, which usually begins at **puberty**. It is characterised by the appearance of **comedones**, **papules**, **pustules** and, in extreme cases, **nodules** and **cysts** on the skin. Red or dark marks may be present from recently healed pustules. It is an abnormal response in the skin to the normal levels of the male hormone **testosterone**, and it affects the areas with the densest number of sebaceous glands: the face, the upper part of the back and the chest. Acne occurs when an excessive amount of *sebum* is produced and dead skin cells accumulate in the *follicle*, thus blocking the mouth of the follicle and trapping the sebum below. In this environment the propionibacterium (a bacterium present on the skin and associated with causing acne) multiplies and *white blood cells* are produced to counteract *infection*. This causes *inflammation* and is characterised by a red papule, which then turns into a pustule, nodule or cyst.

Acromegaly – *ak-r-oh-meg-a-lee* – a condition of the *endocrine system* caused by an over-*secretion* of growth hormone (GH) by the *pituitary gland*. It is a chronic disease characterised by enlargement of the bones of the head, the soft part of the feet and hands, and there may also be enlargement of body organs including the liver, spleen, heart and kidneys. The most serious consequences of this condition are *diabetes mellitus*, *hypertension* and increased risk of *cardiovascular* disease. An excess of *adrenocorticotrophic hormone* (ACTH) may also be produced, affecting the adrenal *cortex* (see *adrenal gland*), which stimulates the production of an excess of *androgens*. This can in turn lead to *hirsutism*.

Acrylic nails – *ak-ril-ik nay-l-s* – false nail *extensions* made from acrylic powder and a liquid, applied over a plastic tip or a nail form (mould). Also known as *sculptured nails*.

Actin – *ak-tin* – a *protein* in *muscle* fibres that helps to contract (shorten and thicken) the muscle and produce movement.

Actinic keratosis – *ak-tin-ik ke-rat-toe-sis* – a pre-cancerous growth that develops from reccuring sun damage and looks like a scaly or crusty bump on the skin. It may vary in colour from dark tan to flesh colour and ranges in size from pinhead size to an inch across. It is most likely to appear on sun-exposed areas such as face, ears, bald scalp, neck, backs of hands and forearms. Also known as solar keratosis.

Activator – *ak-tiv-ay-tor* – something that sets something else in motion or causes a reaction, such as a liquid added to a powder to form an active paste. For example, a liquid *(continued)* activator may be added to a powder *enzyme* to form a mask for the face or a body treatment or rosewater may be added to calamine powder to form a face mask.

Active electrode – *ak-tiv e-lek-tr-oh-d* – the working *electrode* applied to the face or body in *electrotherapy*, through which the electric current flows. In facial *iontophoresis* the active electrodes are the rollers that are used during treatment. In body *faradic treatment* the round graphite pads are placed on a muscle to produce a *contraction* when the current is applied.

Adapting treatment – *ad-ap-tin-g tr-ee-t-men-t* – changing or altering the way in which a *treatment* is carried out to suit a specific condition or purpose and to meet the needs of the *client*.

Add-on treatment – *ad on tr-ee-t-men-t* – an additional *treatment* that complements or links with another.

Addison's disease – *ad–is-ens dis-ee-s* – a *disorder* of the *endocrine system* caused when the *adrenal glands* do not produce enough *cortisol* or *aldosterone*. The disease is characterised by weight loss,

Active listening – *ak-tiv lis-t-n-ing* – an important skill for a *beauty therapist* to practise, particularly when carrying out a *consultation*. It involves the listener paying undivided attention to the speaker and remembering what has been said. A good active listener must focus on the speaker, avoid distractions, be patient, not interrupt, restate points to clarify, ask questions to build understanding, use positive non-verbal gestures and empathise with the speaker.

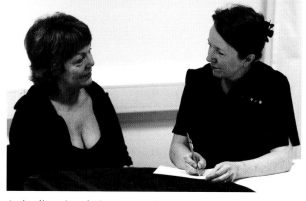

Active listening during a consultation

muscle weakness, fatigue, low blood pressure and sometimes darkening of the skin.

Additive – *ad-it-iv* – a substance added to another to improve it.

Additional – *ad-ish-on-al* – something that is extra, supplementary or added on.

Adduction – *a-duk-shon* – movement of a limb towards the *midline* of the body.

Adductors – *a-duk-t-or-s* – a group of *muscles* in the thigh that include the adductor magnus, the adductor longus, the adductor brevis, the gracilis and the pectineus. They originate from the pelvic bone and attach at intervals along the *femur*. Their function is to move the leg in towards the *midline* of the body and to stabilise the hip joint.

Adenosine triphosphate (ATP) – *ad-en-o-sen tr-eye-fos-f-ay-t* – a major source of energy stored in cells and used to produce *muscle contractions*.

Adhesive – *add-hee-siv* – glue, paste or other sticky substance designed to stick things together.

Adipose tissue – *add-ee-p-oh-s tis-you* – loose *connective tissue* in which fat cells (adipocytes) accumulate. Its main role is to store energy in the form of fat. It is located beneath the skin in the *subcutaneous layer* and around internal organs to provide protective padding. Most adipose tissue is white and its functions are heat insulation, providing a source of energy and cushioning the body. Brown adipose tissue is present in newborn babies, making up about 5% of total body weight and generating essential body heat. Brown adipose tissue diminishes with age to virtually disappear in adulthood.

Adrenal gland – *ad-ree-nal gl-and* – an *endocrine gland*. There are two adrenal glands, one on top of each kidney. Each gland consists of the *medulla* (centre of the *gland*) surrounded by the *cortex* (outer region). The adrenal gland is responsible for regulating the body's *stress* response. The medulla produces *adrenaline* and noradrenaline (a stress *hormone*) and the cortex produces *cortisol* and *aldosterone*, as well (continued)

5

as some sex hormones regulating *metabolism*, sexual function, water balance and stress.

Adrenaline – *ad-ren-a-lin* – a *hormone* produced by the *adrenal glands* that is released into the bloodstream in times of fear and stress. It raises blood sugar levels and stimulates the *nervous system* and the *circulatory system*, increasing the heart rate and blood flow to *muscles*. It suppresses (holds back) the *immune system* and causes the pupils of the eyes to dilate (get bigger), preparing the body for fight or flight. Also known as epinephrine.

Adrenocorticotrophic hormone (ACTH) – *ad-ree-no-kor-tik-oh-trof-ik h-or-m-oh-n* – a *hormone* produced by the *anterior* (front part) *pituitary gland* (which is situated at the base of the brain). It stimulates the adrenal *cortex* (see *adrenal gland*) to release several hormones, including *cortisol*.

Adrenogenital syndrome – *ad-ree-no-jen-it-al sin-dr-oh-m* – a condition affecting both males and females. It results in under-production of the *hormones* *cortisol* and *aldosterone* and

over-production of *androgen*, resulting in early or inappropriate appearance of male characteristics.

Adverse reaction – *ad-ver-s ree-ak-shon* – a possibly harmful or irritating reaction that occurs in response to a stimulus (something that causes a response) such as a product applied to the skin. If this occurs, *treatment* should be stopped immediately, the offending substance removed and a cold compress applied to the area. If the reaction continues the client should be *advised* to seek medical advice.

Advise – *ad-v-eye-z* – to offer an opinion, suggestion or recommendation. *Aftercare*, *home care* and *lifestyle* advice should be provided at the end of each treatment, to support the good effects achieved.

Aerobics – *air-r-oh-bix* – any sustained (continuous) rhythmic exercise (e.g. walking, skipping, jogging, swimming or dancing) that uses the large muscle groups and increases the efficiency of the *circulatory* and *respiratory* *systems*, improving the body's use of oxygen.

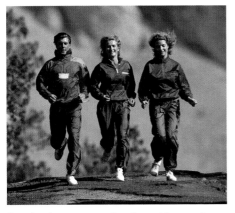

Jogging is one example of aerobic exercise

Aerosol – *air-r-oh-sol* – liquid sealed in a pressurised container which is released as a fine spray through a tiny nozzle.

Aesthetic medicine – *ay-s-th-et-ik med-is-in* – the use of specialised products and equipment to *enhance* the appearance, e.g. improve skin texture, reduce scars and blemishes and leave skin looking more youthful. Products such as *collagen* and *Botox*®, and equipment such as *laser* and *intense pulsed light* (IPL) are used. These *treatments* should be administered only by a medical professional within the scope of their practice.

Afferent – *af-er-rent* – a vessel (channel) or *nerve* that carries a substance or impulse (signal) towards another part of the body. Afferent *lymph vessels* carry *lymph* towards the *lymph nodes* and afferent nerves carry *sensory impulses* (signals to do with the five senses) from the sensory nerves and the sense organs (eyes, ears, etc.) towards the *central nervous system*.

Aftercare advice – *af-t-ker ad-v-eye-s* – recommendations and information provided after a treatment to ensure that the good results are maintained.

Ageing skin – *ay-jin-g sk-in* – skin that shows evidence of dryness, wrinkles, reduced *elasticity* and *muscle tone*, *hyperpigmentation* and change in texture and thickness. The way the skin ages may be chronological (due to normal ageing), *genetic* (determined by inherited factors) or environmental (the result of damage caused by *ultraviolet radiation* and *lifestyle* factors such as smoking, drinking or pollution).

Age spots – *ay-j s-pot-s* – collections of pigment caused by prolonged exposure to the sun or previous sunburn. They are more common in people over the age of 55. They occur on the *(continued)*

7

backs of the hands and other sun-exposed areas such as the face, shoulders, back, arms and feet. Also known as liver spots or solar *lentigo*.

AIDS (acquired immunodeficiency syndrome) – ay-d-s – a condition that develops as a result of infection by *HIV* (human immunodeficiency virus), which attacks the *immune system*, reducing the ability of the body to fight *infection* and leading to possibly life-threatening illnesses.

Aim – ay-m – a purpose, goal or intention, towards which personal effort is directed.

Albino – al-bee-no – a person with no *pigment* in their eyes, hair or skin.

Aldosterone – al-dos-t-r-oh-n – a *hormone* secreted by the *adrenal glands* that regulates the balance of sodium and potassium in the blood.

Algae – al-g-ee – various types of simple organisms containing *chlorophyll* (the green colour in leaves and plants). More commonly referred to as seaweed, algae range in size from single cells to giant kelp and are found mainly in the sea and in tidal pools. They are used for their therapeutic effects in body *treatments*, e.g. as a *diuretic*, for deep cleansing or energy boosting, as an *antioxidant* and to counteract *stress*.

Alkaline – al-ka-l-eye-n – a substance with a *pH* greater than 7, used to neutralise acids and as a base ingredient in many beauty products.

Alkalinity – al-kal-in-it-ee – the state of being *alkaline*. Also the measurement of how alkaline a substance is. Alkalinity is measured on the *pH* scale and alkalis have pH values above 7.

Allantoin – al-an-t-oh-in – a botanical (from a plant) extract from the comfrey plant. It speeds up the natural replacement of body cells, helps to promote the swift healing of damaged or injured tissues and is an effective anti-irritant (reduces *irritation*).

Allergen – *al-er-jen* – a substance, usually eaten or *inhaled*, that causes an *allergic* reaction. Dust, pollen, perfume and peanuts are common allergens.

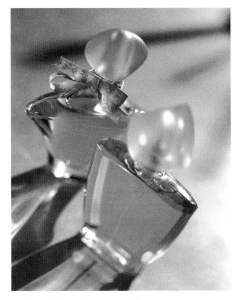

Perfumed products sometimes cause an allergic reaction

Allergic – *al-er-jik* – being sensitive to particular ingredients, products or substances and reacting badly to contact with them. Reactions may include sneezing, wheezing, difficulty breathing, a blocked nose, watery eyes, *hives*, itching, swelling, *erythema*, weakness, dizziness and, in severe cases, *anaphylaxis*.

Allergy – *al-er-jee* – an abnormal reaction of the body's tissues in response to contact with a normally harmless substance. The contact could be through touch or by *inhaling*, eating or drinking the substance. Common symptoms of allergy are sneezing, an itchy, runny or blocked nose, watery eyes, swelling of the eyelids, inflamed skin, *rash*, swelling or blistering skin. More severe reactions include tight chest, *asthma*, *eczema* and, in extreme cases, *anaphylaxis*.

Almond oil – *ol-mon-d oy-l* – oil extracted from the nut of the almond tree. It has a slight odour and a nutty taste and contains vitamins A, B and E. It is used as a *carrier* oil in *aromatherapy*, as an active ingredient in *face masks* (to form a paste when mixed with other substances) and as an *emollient* in facial and body *treatments*.

Aloe vera – *a-lo vee-ra* – a plant native to the Mediterranean. The juice extracted from its fleshy leaves is used for its soothing and healing effects in many cosmetic preparations.

9

Alopecia – *a-lo-pee-sha* – hair loss or baldness, ranging from a small bald patch on the head to loss of all hair over the entire body. The types of alopecia are: androgenetic (hereditary); areata (occurring in patches); barbae (in the beard area); dynamica (baldness resulting from destruction of the *hair follicles*); malign (affecting the entire head including the scalp, eyebrows and beard); mechanica (resulting from the forceful removal of hair or the breaking of hair shafts, e.g. plucking or pulling the hair); senilis (natural hair loss that occurs in older people); and universalis (total loss of hair all over the body).

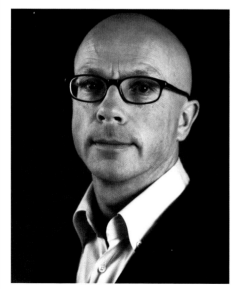

Alopecia

Alpha hydroxy acids (AHA) – *al-fa h-eye-drok-see a-sid-s* – chemical compounds that occur naturally and are used extensively in skin care products. It is claimed that they reduce the signs of ageing and improve the look and texture of the skin. They loosen and dissolve dead skin cells, help to generate new cells, control *acne*, smooth rough, dry skin and improve the texture of sun-damaged and *ageing skin*. *Glycolic acid* is the most widely used AHA. It is manufactured from sugar cane and considered to be the most effective. Other acids are: *lactic acid* from milk, which is milder and less irritating to the skin; citric acid from citrus fruits; malic acid from apples and pears; and tartaric acid from grapes. *Sunscreen* should always be applied immediately after use as the skin will be more sensitive to the damaging effects of *ultraviolet radiation* from the sun.

Alternating current (AC) – *ol-ter-nay-tin-g ku-rent* – an electric current that reverses the direction in a circuit at regular intervals. This is the form in which electricity is delivered to homes and businesses.

Alveolus – *al-vee-oh-lus* (plural **alveoli** – *al-vee-oh-lee*) – the alveoli are the final branches of the *respiratory system*. They are tiny, thin-walled, inflatable sacs (pouches) at the end of the *bronchioles* (the small air passages in the lungs). The *exchange* of gases takes place in the alveoli: oxygen is *inhaled* and absorbed into (taken into) the bloodstream through the thin walls of the alveoli, and carbon dioxide diffuses (passes) from the blood into the alveoli and is then *exhaled*.

Ambience – *am-bee-on-s* – the mood or atmosphere in a particular environment.

Amenorrhoea – *am-en-or-ee-a* – absence of *menstruation*. This may occur as a result of a disorder of the *endocrine system*.

Amino acids – *am-ee-no a-sids* – the basic structural building units of *proteins*. Amino acids form short polymer chains (chemical compounds) called peptides or polypeptides, which in turn form proteins. Combinations of amino acids produce all the proteins that are essential for the *homeostasis* of the human body.

In skin care products, amino acids work as water-binding agents (help the skin to retain moisture) and *antioxidants* and have healing properties.

Ampere – *am-pair* – a unit measuring the strength of electric current, often shortened to *amp*.

Ampoule – *am-p-yoo-l* – a sealed glass or plastic container used for biologically active concentrates that are kept fresh and active until the ampoule is opened for use.

Anabolism – *an-ab-o-lis-m* – the process in which larger *molecules* are built from smaller ones in living matter. It is the first stage of *metabolism* and is necessary for growth, maintenance and *tissue* repair. For example, it increases *muscle* mass and bone growth.

Anaemia – *an-ee-mee-a* – insufficient *haemoglobin* in the blood, often accompanied by a reduction in the number of red blood cells. It may cause weakness, breathlessness and paleness of the skin.

Anaerobics – *an-er-r-oh-bix* – the opposite of *aerobic* exercise. It consists of short-duration, high-intensity, strength-based activity such as weightlifting or bodybuilding. Anaerobic means 'without oxygen' – this refers to the fact that the muscles do not receive enough oxygen to carry out the activity so they have to produce energy in another way that doesn't depend on oxygen.

Anagen – *an-a-jen* – the active growth phase of a *hair follicle* during which the hair is fully attached to the blood supply, hair cells grow rapidly, producing the *hair shaft* from the follicle, which itself grows deeper into the skin.

Analyse – *an-a-l-eye-s* – to study or examine something in detail in order to discover more about it.

Analysis – *an-al-i-sis* – an investigation of information or facts. An analysis may involve several different parts. For example, the therapist asks the client questions during consultation to gain useful information for planning the most appropriate treatment. Client record cards provide additional useful, up-to-date information concerning previous treatments, medical history, **lifestyle**, **home care advice**, **contraindications**, **contra-actions** and **modifications to treatment**. A visual analysis is also carried out by closely inspecting the client's skin, nail, hair or body condition before treatment is planned.

Anaphoresis – *an-a-for-ee-sis* – the movement of negatively charged *ions* towards the *anode* (the positive *electrode*).

Anaphylaxis – *an-a-fill-ax-is* – a severe, sometimes life-threatening *allergic* reaction that occurs within minutes of exposure to an offending substance. Chemicals such as *histamine* that are involved in *immune system* reactions can produce serious skin symptoms, such as *hives* and swelling, as well as severe breathing problems. They also produce a dramatic widening of the *blood vessels*, which results in a rapid drop in *blood pressure*.

Anatomy – *an-at-o-mee* – the study of the structure and organisation of living things. Human anatomy is the study of bodily structure, bones, *muscles*, organs and all body systems including *circulatory*, *digestive*, *endocrine*, *immune*, *integumentary*, *lymphatic*, *muscular*, *nervous*, *reproductive*, *respiratory*, *skeletal* and *excretory*.

Androgens – *and-ro-jens* – *hormones* that control the development of male characteristics and that cause abnormal hair growth in women.

Angioma – *an-jee-o-ma* – a *benign tumour* made up of small *blood vessels*. It usually appears at or near the surface of the skin. A cherry angioma is the most common, also called senile angioma. It is made of clusters of tiny *capillaries* ranging in colour from bright red to purple. As it grows it forms a dome shape. A spider angioma occurs just beneath the surface of the skin. It contains a central red spot with tiny red lines extending from it that resemble spider legs.

Anhidrosis – *an-h-eye-dr-oh-sis* – lack of perspiration (sweating).

Anion – *an-eye-on* – a negatively charged *ion* that is attracted to the *anode* (the positive *electrode*).

Anode – *an-oh-d* – the positive pole or *electrode*.

Anorexia nervosa – *an-or-rex-ee-a ner-v-oh-sa* – a disorder characterised by loss of appetite and bizarre eating patterns, which can result in excessive weight loss. The weight loss is caused by avoiding fattening foods, refusing to eat, excessive exercise, use of laxatives or *diuretics* or self-induced vomiting. Sufferers are preoccupied with the size and shape of their body and have an overwhelming fear of putting on weight. The weight loss may cause hormonal imbalance and women with this condition may stop menstruating (having monthly periods).

Antagonist – *an-tag-on-is-t* – a *muscle* that has the opposite action to another muscle, e.g. the *biceps* and the *triceps*.

Anterior – *an-tee-ree-or* – the front surface or at the front. Also known as ventral.

Anti-ageing – *an-tee ay-jin-g* – literally means 'against ageing'. Products or **treatments** that are described as anti-ageing are designed to combat the effects of ageing or to defend the skin and body against the ageing process.

Antibacterial – *an-tee-bak-tee-ree-al* – describes an ingredient that destroys or prevents the growth of **bacteria**.

Antibiotic – *an-tee-by-ot-ik* – a drug that kills or prevents the growth of **bacteria**.

Antibody – *an-tee-bod-ee* – a chemical produced by **white blood cells** to neutralise or destroy **antigens**, **bacteria**, **viruses** and other foreign bodies (objects coming from outside the body).

Antidiuretic hormone (ADH) – *an-tee-die-or-ret-ik hor-m-oh-n* – a **hormone** produced by the **hypothalamus** and released by the **pituitary gland** when the body is low on water. It causes the kidneys to reabsorb more water (see **absorption**). Also known as vasopressin.

Antifungal – *an-tee-fun-g-l* – destroying or preventing the growth of **fungi**.

Antigen – *an-tee-jen* – a substance or foreign body (object coming from outside the body) that can stimulate the production of **antibodies**.

Anti-inflammatory – *an-tee-in-f-lam-a-t-ree* – an ingredient that reduces signs of **inflammation** such as redness, swelling, tenderness, pain or **irritation**.

Antioxidants – *an-tee-ox-id-ants* – biochemicals (substances produced by chemical reactions in living organisms) that slow down the damaging effect of **free radicals**. **Vitamins** A, C and E are powerful antioxidants. Eating plenty of fruit and vegetables such as carrots, squash, broccoli, peppers, tomatoes, peaches, apricots, blueberries, citrus fruits, strawberries and nuts, seeds and whole grains helps to ensure that the body is supplied with sufficient antioxidants.

Antiseptic – *an-tee-sep-tik* – a chemical agent that inhibits (prevents or hinders) the growth and reproduction of *bacteria* and other harmful micro-organisms (microscopic organisms).

Aorta – *ay-or-t-a* – the main *artery* of the *circulatory system*, with the largest diameter and the thickest walls. It carries oxygenated blood (blood with a high concentration of oxygen) from the left *ventricle* of the heart to smaller arteries and *capillaries* which carry the blood to the *tissues* of the body.

Apocrine glands – *a-po-k-ree-n g-l-an-s* – *sweat glands* that occur on hairy parts of the body, especially the armpits and groin. They develop during *puberty* and produce *sweat* that contains fatty materials. Body odour is caused by *bacteria* breaking down the organic compounds in the sweat.

Aponeurosis – *ap-oh-n-you-r-oh-sis* – a sheet-like layer of *connective tissue* joining one *muscle* with another or with bone.

Appearance – *a-pee-er-an-s* – how somebody looks, outward show.

Appendage – *a-pen-dij* – something added or attached to something larger.

Appendicular skeleton – *ay-pen-dik-you-la sk-el-e-t-n* – the bones of the skeleton that make up the *shoulder girdle*, the *pelvic girdle* and the upper and lower limbs (arms and legs). (See the diagram on page 195.)

Appendix – *a-pen-dik-s* – a small projection (outgrowth) of lymphoid tissue (tissue that fights infection) in the intestine on the lower right-hand side of the body.

Applicator – *a-p-lik-ay-tor* – a simple device for applying a substance, e.g. a brush used to apply a *face mask* to the skin.

Appointment – *ap-oy-n-t-men-t* – a time reserved for a *treatment* in a salon or for a meeting or social engagement.

Appraisal – *ap-rays-l* – the assessment or judgement of an individual based on their performance, or an estimate of something's value.

Apricot kernel oil – *ay-p-rik-cot ker-n-l oy-l* – a fine- *(continued)* textured *carrier oil* used in *aromatherapy*. It is easily absorbed by the skin and especially good for massage of the face.

Aquaerobics – *a-kwa-r-oh-bix* – exercise using water resistance to strengthen and tone *muscles*.

Aqueous – *a-kwee-us* – anything relating to, similar to, dissolved in or containing water.

Aroma – *a-r-oh-m-a* – a distinctive smell or fragrance.

Aromatherapy – *a-r-oh-ma-th-e-rap-ee* – the use of fragrance to alter or affect a person's mood, behaviour or well-being. *Essential oils* are extracted from plants – flowers, leaves, bark, wood, roots, seeds, herbs and peel – and may be used for therapeutic effects, e.g. to promote relaxation. They can be blended with a *carrier oil* to provide massage, added to facial and body care products or diffused in an essential oil burner. Essential oils may also be incorporated into pot pourri or candles to fragrance a room, as well as into air fresheners, compresses or floral waters.

Aromatherapy massage – *a-r-oh-ma-th-e-rap-ee mas-ar-j* – *essential oils* are blended with a *carrier oil* and used to provide a massage treatment.

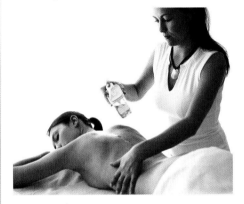

An aromatherapy massage

Arrector pili muscles – *a-rek-t-or pil-eye m-us-el* – fan-shaped *smooth muscles* in the *dermis*. An arrector pili muscle is attached to the base of each hair. It contracts when the body surface is chilled, causing the hair to stand erect (straight up).

Arteriole – *ar-tee-ree-oh-l* – a small branch of an *artery* that delivers blood to the *capillaries*.

Arteriosclerosis – *ar-tee-ree-oh-sk-l-er-oh-sis* – a gradual deterioration (worsening of physical condition) in the *arteries* characterised by thickening of the walls and a build-up of calcium. It causes a loss of *elasticity* and restricts blood flow through the artery.

Artery – *ar-t-er-ee* (plural **Arteries** – *ar-t-er-ees*) – the largest of the *blood vessels* that carry blood away from the heart, with thick, muscular walls. They branch into *arterioles* and then *capillaries*.

Arthritis – *ar-th-r-eye-tis* – *inflammation* of the *joints* that causes pain and/or difficulty in moving about. The most common types are rheumatoid arthritis and osteoarthritis.

Artificial lashes – *ar-tif-ish-l lash-z* – semi-permanent individual lashes or temporary strip lashes that are applied to the natural lashes to make them appear longer or thicker. The latest trend is for eyelash *extensions* – a special bonding agent is used to apply the false lash directly to the real lash.

Artificial nails – *ar-tif-ish-l nay-l-z* – false nails may be either temporary – applied with glue to the natural nail – or semi-permanent – applied using a special system such as *acrylic* or *gel nails*.

Asepsis – *ay-sep-sis* – absence of *pathogenic* (harmful) *bacteria*.

Aseptic – *ay-sep-tik* – free from *infection* and organisms that cause *disease*.

Asian skin – *ay-sh-on s-kin* – this skin type originates from Japan, China, the Middle East, India, Pakistan, Sri Lanka and Malaysia. The depth of colour varies from the paler-skinned light Oriental to very dark Asian. The lighter shades have yellow undertones as there is *(continued)*

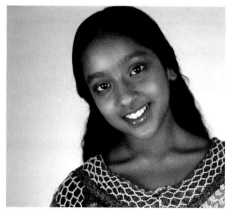

Asian skin types include Indian and Oriental

more carotene (orange-yellow *pigment*) present in the **stratum corneum**. The darker shades have more eumelanin (a brown pigment containing **melanin**) present. Problems may vary, e.g. darker pigmented areas of skin or **keloid** scars. In general, skin types include normal, dry, oily and sensitive, depending on environmental conditions, skin care and diet.

Assimilation – *a-sim-il-ay-shon* – the conversion of foods that have been absorbed into the bloodstream into living *tissue*.

Assistance – *as-is-tan-s* – help, aid or support provided by one individual to another.

Association – *as-oh-see-ay-shon* – an organised group of people who have an activity or purpose in common. Professional associations are useful as they provide help and advice, as well as insurance and training opportunities that will help in *continuing professional development*.

Asteatosis – *as-tee-a-t-oh-sis* – a condition characterised by low amounts or a complete lack of *sebum* produced by the **sebaceous glands**, causing dry skin conditions.

Asthma – *a-s-th-ma* – a *respiratory* disorder caused by *allergies* that constrict (narrow) the **bronchioles**, cause spasms (violent *contractions*) in the muscles surrounding the lungs and cause the bronchioles to swell or clog them with mucus (a slimy fluid).

Astringent – *a-strin-jen-t* – a substance that dries or tightens the surface to which it is applied. It is used to remove surface grease from the skin and to tighten the pores and is an ingredient of a clay **face mask** for *oily skin*.

Atherosclerosis – *a-th-e-r-oh-sk-l-er-oh-sis* – a form of *arteriosclerosis* in which a fatty substance (known as plaque) builds up on the inner walls of the *arteries*.

Athlete's foot – *a-th-lee-t-s fut* – a fungal *infection* that affects the spaces between the toes. It is moist and white in appearance, and there may be some scaling of the skin. It is usually itchy and there may be some *inflammation*. It is caused by harmless *parasites* on the skin called dermatophytes, which feed on dead skin cells. It is a common infection that flourishes in warm, moist conditions and can affect anyone, particularly people who wear tight-fitting shoes, do not dry their feet properly or sweat excessively. It is contagious (spread by contact) and can be spread directly through skin-to-skin contact or indirectly. Also known as *tinea pedis*.

Atom – *a-t-m* – a tiny unit of matter, consisting of a *nucleus*, neutrons, protons and *electrons*.

Atomise – *a-t-m-eyes* – to reduce to a fine spray or tiny particles.

Atrium – *ay-tree-um (plural Atria* – ay-tree-a) – the atria are the two upper chambers (right and left) of the heart that receive blood from the *veins* and force it into the *ventricles*.

Atrophy – *a-t-r-oh-fee* – wasting away or decreasing in size, e.g. loss of strength and size

of muscles after being in a plaster cast.

Atrophic scar – *ay-trof-ik s-k-ar* – a scar that is lower than the surrounding tissue, causing a dent in the skin.

Audiosonic – *or-dee-oh-son-ik* – a hand-held sound wave vibrator used to gently massage body *tissues*. Deeply penetrating sound waves are transmitted to an area through a small *applicator* and may penetrate as far as 6 centimetres, relieving tension in tightly contracted muscles.

Authorisation – *or-th-or-eye-say-shon* – official permission or approval.

Autoclave – *or-t-oh-cl-ay-v* – equipment used to *sterilise* small metal instruments using steam under pressure.

Autoimmune disease – *or-t-oh-im-you-n d-is-ees* – a disease that results when the immune system mistakenly attacks the body's own tissues, e.g. *multiple sclerosis*, type 1 *diabetes*, rheumatoid *arthritis* and systemic lupus (a chronic condition *(continued)*

19

in which antibodies attack the body's connective tissues).

Autonomic nervous system – or-t-oh-nom-ik n-er-v-us sis-t-m – the part of the *peripheral nervous system* that controls the automatic activity of many organs and *muscles* in the body and is responsible for *homeostasis*. It is divided into the *sympathetic* and *parasympathetic nervous systems*.

Avocado oil – a-vo-kar-d-oh oy-l – a *carrier oil* used in *aromatherapy*. It is suitable for facial massage and treating *mature skin*.

Axial skeleton – ax-ee-al s-kel-e-t-n – the part of the skeleton that forms the central axis of the body, consisting of the skull, the vertebral column (spine), the *ribs* and the *sternum*. (See the diagram on page 195.)

Axilla – ax-ill-a – the armpit.

Axillary glands – ax-ill-a-ree g-l-and-s – *lymph nodes* situated under the arm, next to the breast area, that receive *lymph drainage* from the arms, *shoulder girdle*

and mammary glands (breasts). (See the diagram on page 199.)

Axon – ax-on – the part of a *neuron* that carries an impulse (signal) away from the body of the cell.

Ayurveda – eye-y-vay-d – the ancient Hindu science of health and medicine using herbal treatments and hot oils, combined with meditation, nutrition and aromatherapy, to create an overall balance of self. The Ayurvedic body functions, called *doshas*, consist of: Vata, referring to blood, circulation and healing; Pitta, referring to heat and *metabolism*; and Kapha, the structure of the spiritual and philosophical self.

Ayurvedic massage – eye-y-vay-d-ik ma-s-ar-j – similar to *Swedish massage*, but with specially formulated fragrant oils, mixed to match a client's *doshas*.

Azulene – as-y-oo-lee-n – a substance extracted from chamomile and yarrow flowers. It is an *anti-inflammatory* and helps soothe the skin.

Bacteria – *bak-tee-ree-a* – single-celled micro-organisms (microscopic organisms) that are found everywhere. They can be either *pathogenic* (capable of causing disease) or non-pathogenic (not capable of causing disease).

Bactericidal – *bak-tee-ri-s-eye-d-al* – capable of killing *bacteria*.

Bactericide – *bak-tee-ri-s-eye-d* – an agent used to kill germs.

Balinese massage – *ba-lin-ees mas-ar-j* – an ancient massage technique passed down through generations of families in Bali, Indonesia. It combines a variety of massage techniques, including deep tissue massage, acupressure and gentle stretches. It stimulates the flow of blood, oxygen and *qi* (energy) around the body to promote relaxation, reduce stress, rebalance the body and soothe aching joints and muscles.

Balneotherapy – *bal-nee-oh-th-e-rap-ee* – therapeutic bathing, the use of water to restore or revitalise the body by improving circulation, reducing *stress*, speeding up cell activity and boosting the *immune system*.

Treatments include bathing in hot water springs and mineral-rich waters, either the whole body or in small baths for areas such as the feet.

Basal cell carcinoma – *bay-s-l sell car-sin-o-ma* – a skin cancer that starts in the *epidermis*. It is slow growing and painless and usually appears on areas of the skin that are regularly exposed to sunlight. It is characterised by new skin growth that bleeds easily or does not heal. If left untreated, it may grow into surrounding tissues and bone. Also known as a rodent ulcer.

Basal layer – *bay-s-l lay-r* – see *stratum germinativum*.

Base coat – *bay-s k-oh-t* – the first coat of enamel applied to the *nail plate* at the end of a *manicure* or *pedicure*, to protect the nail from staining, to prolong the life of the enamel or for other beneficial effects such as strengthening or hydrating (moisturising) the nail.

Basophils – *bay-so-fils* – white granular blood cells formed in bone marrow (soft tissue in the centre of bones) that *(continued)* produce *histamine* when they are stimulated. They leave the blood and accumulate at the site of *infection* or *inflammation* and contribute to the inflammatory reaction.

Beau's lines – *b-oh-s l-eye-n-s* – grooves or lines that run across the nail plate. They may be due to trauma (injury or shock), illness, malnutrition or skin disease and are the result of an interruption in the *protein* formation of the *nail plate*.

Beauty – *b-you-tee* – a quality or feature that looks attractive and gives pleasure.

Beauty therapist – *b-you-tee th-e-rap-is-t* – a person who provides beauty and holistic therapies in a salon, *spa* or other beauty establishment.

Beeswax – *bee-s-wa-ks* – a solid, yellow substance produced by bees to construct their honeycombs. It is used to make candles and skin care products.

Benefits – *ben-e-fit-s* – advantages, features that will make an improvement or *enhance* well-being. Describing the benefits of treatments and products is an important part of making a sale, as the end result is what interests the client most when making a decision.

Benign – *be-n-eye-n* – not *malignant*, of no danger to health.

Benzocaine – *ben-zo-kay-n* – a drug used as a local anaesthetic (substance that causes loss of feeling).

Beta hydroxy acid – *be-ta h-eye-dr-ox-ee a-sid* – a skin *exfoliant* similar to *alpha hydroxy acid*. It is oil-soluble (dissolves in oil), which allows it to penetrate into the opening of the *hair follicle* and exfoliate the dead skin cells that have accumulated. This makes it particularly effective on *acne*-prone skin. It is derived from aspirin, which has *anti-inflammatory* properties, so it is less irritating to the skin than alpha hydroxy acid, making it more suitable for a *sensitive skin*. *Sunscreen* must be applied immediately after use to protect the skin from damage due to exposure to *ultraviolet radiation*. See also *salycilic acid*.

Biceps – *b-eye-sep-s* – the prominent muscle on the inside of the upper arm. It *flexes* the elbow and rotates the forearm. (See the diagram on page 202.)

Bile – *by-l* – a digestive juice secreted by the liver and stored in the gall bladder. It helps in the digestion of fats.

Bio- – *b-eye-o* – a prefix (beginning part of a word) meaning 'relating to living organisms'.

Blackhead – *b-lak-hed* – see *comedo*.

Bleaching – *bl-ee-ch-in-g* – the removal of colour by means of chemical agents or sunlight.

Blemish – *bl-em-ish* – an imperfection or mark on the skin, e.g. a *scar*, birthmark, *pustule* or *hyperpigmentation*.

Blend epilation – *b-len-d ep-il-ay-shon* – the use of *(continued)*

Black skin – *b-lak s-kin* – this skin type contains cells that are capable of producing large amounts of *melanin*. The amount produced will determine the depth of colour. It has the ability to absorb more *ultraviolet radiation* than lighter skin colours, thus providing increased protection from sunburn, skin cancer and other *lesions* that form in response to exposure to ultraviolet radiation. Ageing effects on the skin are also delayed, *collagen* and *elastin* breakdown is slower, allowing the skin to remain supple and look smoother for longer than other skin types. The *epidermis* is generally thicker, and *sweat glands* and *sebaceous glands* are larger and more numerous. They are situated nearer the skin surface causing large, open pores and an oily appearance. Black skin is more susceptible to the following problems: *keloid* scars, *dermatosis papulosa nigra* and *pseudofolliculitis barbae* in men.

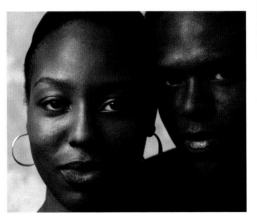

Black skin

direct current and short-wave *diathermy* together, combining the more thorough *galvanic current* (a direct current produced chemically) with the speed of the short-wave diathermy to treat *superfluous* hair.

Blending – b-len-din-g – the technique used to prevent a demarcation line appearing during the application of *makeup*. *Also* a nail art technique which may include the use of opalescent blending or the blending of several colours. *Also* combining *essential oils* with a *carrier oil* in *aromatherapy*.

Blister – b-lis-t-er – a small pocket that forms between the *epidermis* and *dermis* containing serum (a clear, watery fluid) and protecting the tissues underneath. May occur as a result of *sunburn*, *allergic* reaction or injury.

Blocked pores – bl-o-k-d p-or-s – a build-up of *sebum* and dead skin cells in the openings of the *follicles* in the skin. They may become *comedones* (when the sebum oxidises – mixes with oxygen on exposure to the air) or *milia* (when a layer of *epidermal tissue* grows over the follicle opening, protecting the sebum from *oxidisation*).

Blood – b-l-u-d – a liquid *tissue*, a mixture of *plasma* and specialised cells that circulates around the body in *blood vessels*. Red blood cells transport oxygen to the cells, *white blood cells* produce *antibodies* to fight infection and *platelets* help with blood clotting.

Blood glucose – b-l-u-d g-loo-k-oh-s – sugar found in the blood which is the main source of energy for the body.

Blood pressure – b-l-u-d pre-sh-or – the measurement of the force applied to the walls of the *arteries* as the heart pumps blood through the body. Systolic pressure is the maximum pressure in an artery at the moment when the heart is beating and pumping blood through the body. Diastolic pressure is the minimum pressure in an artery in the moments between beats when the heart is resting.

Blood shunting – b-l-u-d sh-un-tin-g – occurs when blood is suddenly re-routed from one part of the body to another to cope with the increased demand. Shortly after exercise begins, blood is shunted to the muscles to cope with the demand. During heat *treatment* such as *sauna* and *steam bath*, blood is shunted to the skin and away from the vital organs to help the body maintain a normal temperature.

Blood spots – b-l-u-d s-pot-s – tiny concentrations of blood on the skin's surface, overlaid with a translucent (almost transparent) layer of skin.

Blood vessels – b-l-u-d ve-s-l-s – channels (*arteries*, *veins* and *capillaries*) that carry blood to and from the heart and body *tissues*. (See the diagram on page 199.)

Blue nails – b-loo n-ay-l-z – may be caused by medical conditions that reduce the amount of oxygen in the blood such as *anaemia*, pulmonary (lung) disease, peripheral arterial disease (which affects the arteries in the pelvis and legs) or as a side effect of some medication.

Blusher – b-lu-sh-er – a type of makeup used to add warmth and shape to the cheeks or to even out skin tone. It comes as powder, *gel*, cream, liquid, mousse or liquid applied with a spray.

Body fat – bod-ee-fat – oily substance produced and stored in the body. When the intake of calories is higher than the body requires for general maintenance and physical activity, the excess is stored as fat. Essential body fat is required for normal body functioning and is stored in bone marrow, the heart, lungs, liver, spleen, kidneys, intestines and muscles. Stored fat is found in *adipose tissue*, mostly beneath the skin in the *subcutaneous layer*, where it provides insulation and cushions the body. It is also found around some internal organs for protection. There are two types of adipose tissue: white fat (which is important in energy *metabolism*, heat insulation and cushioning) and brown fat (which is found mostly in newborn babies and is important for making heat).

Body language – *bod-ee lan-g-w-ij* – a non-verbal form of communication using gestures, facial expressions and *posture* - often done without realising.

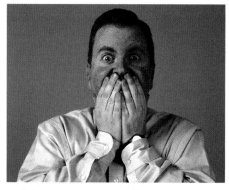

Body language conveys different messages

Body scrub – *bod-ee s-kr-ub* – a type of *exfoliation* treatment used to improve skin texture and to soften and moisturise the skin.

Body wraps – *bod-ee rap-s* – a *spa* or beauty *treatment* in which the body is covered in mud, *algae*, herbs, oils or other products before being wrapped tightly in bandages, linen, plastic, foil or a thermal blanket. The effects are *detoxification*, temporary inch loss and tighter, firmer, softer, cleaner or hydrated skin.

Boil – *boy-l* – a localised (in one place) *infection* deep in the skin.

It begins as a red, tender area of skin and becomes harder, except for the centre, which is soft and filled with pus (a mixture of infection-fighting *white blood cells*, *proteins* and *bacteria*). This eventually forms a head which may be surgically lanced to remove it or it may drain on its own.

Botox® – *b-oh-tox* – the brand name for the non-toxic botulinum *toxin*. It is a neuromuscular (affecting both nerves and muscles) blocking agent. When injected into the muscles, particularly of the face, it prevents movement and causes certain wrinkles to disappear completely. It paralyses the muscle injected by preventing the release of acetylcholine (a substance that helps to transmit nerve impulses in the body) from the *motor nerves*. Without a nerve supply the muscle fibre withers away, until the nerve regenerates (renews itself) and the muscle strengthens again. It is used effectively to treat many medical conditions, such as spasms (repeated *contractions*) of the eyelid, squints, *hyperhidrosis* and some muscular diseases.

Brachioradialis – *brak-ee-oh-rad-ee-ay-lis* – a muscle of the forearm. Its action is to **flex** the elbow at the forearm and assist in **pronation** and **supination**. (See the diagram on page 202.)

British Standards Institution (BSI) – an independent national organisation for the UK whose objectives are to promote health and safety, protect the environment and establish quality standards.

Brittle nails – *br-it-l nay-l-z* – hard, dry and inflexible nails that snap easily. This condition can be caused by exposure to harsh chemicals (products that strip the nail of natural oils), exposure to extreme cold or overuse of nail strengtheners.

Bronchi – *br-on-kee* – tubes that carry air from the trachea (windpipe) to the lungs.

Bronchioles – *br-on-kee-oh-l-s* – small tubes in the lungs that are formed by the branching of the **bronchi**. They terminate in the **alveoli**.

Brow ptosis – *br-ow toe-sis* – a condition where the forehead sags, causing the eyebrows to droop over the eyelids, which then feel heavy. It may be caused by loose skin resulting from ageing, gravity and loss of **collagen** or by underlying fat in the **subcutaneous layer**.

Buccinator – *buk-sin-ay-tor* – a thin, flat **muscle** lining the cheek. It contracts and compresses (squeezes) the cheek against the teeth and retracts (pulls back) the mouth. (See the diagram on page 192.)

Budget – *bud-jit* – a detailed summary of estimated or intended spending for a given period, together with proposals for financing the expenditure.

Buffing – *buff-in-g* – a method used to achieve a high polish on the nails. Suitable for clients who are **allergic** to enamel or who are not allowed to wear it for work. Buffing reduces ridges on the surface of the nail plate and removes stains. Can be used for a male **manicure**.

Buffing paste – *buff-in-g pay-s-t* – a product that can be used when **buffing** nails to remove stains and ridges. It is made from powdered silica or pumice *(continued)* mixed with a combination of wax and mineral oil to form a smooth paste.

Bulimia – *bul-im-ee-a* – a *psychological* eating disorder characterised by uncontrollable overeating or binge eating, followed by forced vomiting or overuse of laxatives.

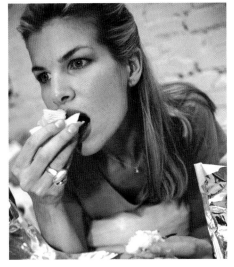

Binge eating is a symptom of bulimia

Bunion – *bun-yon* – an enlargement of bone or tissue around the *joint* at the base of the big toe that causes a bump on the joint. The big toe is often turned inwards towards the second toe and the tissue surrounding the joint may be swollen and tender. Also known as *hallux valgus*.

Bursa – *b-er-sa* – a small sac (pouch), found in *synovial joints*, that is lined with synovial membrane (a thin layer of tissue lining a cavity) and filled with synovial fluid, which acts as a cushion to reduce friction between tendons and bones.

Business plan – *bis-ness pl-an* – a written document that describes a business, the objectives, the market and the expected income and expenditure. A business plan is essential when borrowing money to start or expand a business.

Business status – *bis-ness st-ay-tus* – the legal position or structure of a business, which could be as a *sole trader*, a *partnership* or a *limited company*.

Buying signals – *b-eye-in-g sig-n-l-s* – physical or verbal clues that a client sends out that tell you they are interested in making a purchase.

Byelaw – *b-eye-lor* – a local law relevant to a particular area or an internal rule in a company or organisation.

Calamine – *ka-la-my-n* – a fine mineral powder used as an ingredient in **face masks** and soothing lotions. It calms an itchy skin and is useful for treating **sunburn**, **sensitive skin** and some **rashes**.

Calcaneus – *kal-kay-nee-us* – the bone making up the heel of the foot. (See the diagram on page 197.)

Calcitonin – *kal-si-t-oh-n-in* – a **hormone** produced by the **thyroid gland** that plays a role in controlling calcium levels.

Caldarium – *kal-der-ee-um* – the hottest room in the original Roman baths. Used to detoxify the body after being massaged with oils in the relaxation room.

Callus – *kal-us* – an especially tough area of skin which has become relatively thick due to repeated contact, friction or pressure. Most often found on the hands and feet.

Calorie – *kal-or-ee* – a unit of energy. The amount of energy required to raise the temperature of one gram of water by one degree Celsius.

Camphor – *kam-fer* – an aromatic (scented) **resin** obtained from the wood or leaves of the camphor tree. It is white, translucent (semi-transparent) and used in preparations to relieve pain and mild itching.

Candelilla wax – *kan-del-lee-la wak-s* – used as a thickening agent and **emollient** in lipsticks and stick foundations.

Capacitor – *kap-as-it-or* – an electrical device that stores an electrical charge. Formerly called a **condenser**.

Capillaries – *kap-il-a-ree-s* – the smallest **blood vessels** in the body. They have thin walls and are located between **arterioles** and **venules**. They are one cell thick, allowing the **exchange** of substances such as oxygen, water and lipids (fatty chemicals) between blood cells and body cells.

Carbohydrates – *karb-oh-h-eye-d-ray-t-s* – **molecules** composed of carbon, hydrogen and oxygen that provide energy and structural materials for cells in the body. They are contained in foods such as bread, rice, pasta, potatoes and sugar.

Carbon dioxide – *kar-bon-d-eye-oks-eye-d* – a colourless, odourless (with no smell), incombustible (not capable of burning) gas, present in the atmosphere. It is produced by cell *metabolism* and is eliminated from the body when *exhaling*.

Cardiac – *kar-dee-ak* – relating to the heart.

Cardiac cycle – *kar-dee-ak s-eye-kl* – one complete heartbeat, consisting of one contraction and relaxation of the atria and one contraction and relaxation of the ventricles.

Cardiac muscle – *kar-dee-ak mus-sel* – a specialised form of striated (striped) *involuntary muscle* in the heart. (See the diagram on page 198.)

Cardio- – *kar-dee-oh* – a prefix (beginning part of a word) meaning relating to the heart.

Cardiovascular – *kar-dee-oh-vas-q-lar* – relating to the *circulatory system* (the heart and the *blood vessels*).

Cardiovascular system – *kar-dee-oh-vas-q-lar sis-t-m* – see *circulatory system*.

Carmine – *kar-my-n* – a natural red colour that comes from the dried female cochineal beetle, used to colour lip gloss, lipstick and other cosmetics.

Carpals – *kar-pulls* – the bones that make up the wrist *joint*, consisting of the hamate, capitate, pisiform, triquetral, lunate, scaphoid, trapezium and trapezoid. (See the diagram on page 197.)

Carrier oil – *ka-ree-er oy-l-s* – a liquid used to dilute *essential oils* before applying them to the skin. They provide the necessary lubricant (slippery substance) for an *aromatherapy* massage. Different carrier oils have different effects. They are generally cold-pressed vegetable oils. They do not evaporate (unlike essential oils) and they have very little aroma. Some popular carrier oils include sweet almond, grapeseed, avocado, olive, sesame and evening primrose oils. Also known as a base oil.

Cartilage – *kar-til-aj* – a firm, flexible, elastic type of **connective tissue** found in various parts of the body.

Cash – *k-a-sh* – money in the form of coins and banknotes used to make purchases.

Cash equivalents – *k-ash ek-wiv-a-lent-s* – items used instead of cash to make a payment – e.g. cheques, credit and debit cards, gift vouchers and discount vouchers.

Cash flow forecast – *k-ash-flo for-kas-t* – a prediction of all expected business expenses and income over a given period.

Cash point – *k-ash poy-n-t* – the place at which payment is made. *Also* an automated machine that allows financial transactions to take place, e.g. cash withdrawals and deposits.

Catabolism – *kat-a-bol-is-m* – the chemical reactions that break down complex **molecules** into simpler ones for energy production.

Catagen – *kat-a-jen* – the transitional stage in the development of a **hair follicle** after **anagen** and before **telogen**. The papilla separates from the germinal **matrix** (the cells where the hair is formed) and the hair moves up the follicle, the papilla collapses and the lower half of the follicle breaks down. (See the diagram on page 191.)

Cataphoresis – *kat-a-for-ee-sis* – the movement of positively charged **ions** to the **cathode**.

Cathode – *ka-th-oh-d* – the negative pole or **electrode**.

Cation – *kat-i-on* – a positively charged **ion** that is attracted to the **cathode**.

Caustic – *kor-s-tik* – describes a substance that destroys tissue.

Cauterise – *kort-er-eye-s* – to destroy tissue by direct application of heat or a **caustic** agent.

Cell – *sell* – the basic unit of all living things. (See the diagram on page 188.)

Cell membrane – *sell mem-br-ay-n* – the outer layer of a cell composed of lipids (fatty chemicals) and **proteins**. *(continued)*

It is essential for the effective functioning of each cell. It is protective and **semi-permeable**, allowing substances to pass into and out of the cell. (See the diagram on page 188.)

Cellulite – *sel-you-l-eye-t* – fatty tissue causing a dimpled or uneven appearance in the skin of certain parts of the body, mostly in women. It occurs when fat cells swell and the surrounding tissue changes in texture, causing a pulling on the tissues and giving the skin the dimpled effect. It is thought that hormonal changes contribute to the condition, particularly during **puberty** and pregnancy.

Central nervous system – *sen-tr-ul-ner-vus sis-t-em* – the largest part of the **nervous system**, consisting of the brain and spinal cord. Together with the **peripheral nervous system**, it has a role in the control of behaviour. The brain receives sensory (to do with the five senses) information from the spinal cord and its own nerves, it processes this information and then initiates a response. The spinal cord transmits information to the brain and carries information from the brain to the **muscles** and **glands**

of the body. (See the diagram on page 201.)

Ceramides – *se-ram-eye-ds* – lipids (fatty chemicals) that are naturally present in the skin and help to provide a moisture barrier or seal. When ceramides are added to skin care products they help to strengthen this seal, allowing the skin to remain moisturised for longer.

Cerebellum – *se-reb-e-lum* – the part of the brain concerned with fine coordination of body movement, **posture** and balance. It is attached to the brain stem at the base of the brain.

Cerebral cortex – *se-ree-br-l c-or-tex* – the outer layer of grey matter (the active part of the brain) in the **cerebrum**. It is involved in higher brain functions such as language and abstract thought.

Cerebral hemispheres – *se-ree-br-l hem-is-fee-r-s* – the two symmetrical halves of the brain divided by the cerebral fissure. A popular theory is that the right hemisphere controls creativity and emotion and the left hemisphere controls logic, analysis and spatial reasoning.

Cerebrum – *ser-ee-br-um* – the *anterior* (front) and largest part of the brain, consisting of two halves known as hemispheres.

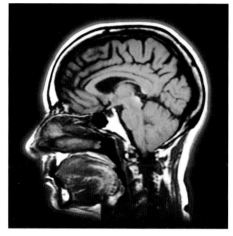

The brain

Chakra – *sh-ak-ra* – an Ayurvedic (see *Ayurveda*) term meaning 'energy centre', used to describe the seven centres of spiritual energy in the human body.

Chamomile or Camomile – *kam-o-my-l* – a flowering plant that has been used since at least the time of the ancient Egyptians for medicinal and therapeutic purposes. It is now a popular *essential oil* in *aromatherapy*

massage for calming and relaxing.

Check – *ch-e-k* – to investigate or verify that information is correct.

Chemical peel – *kem-ik-l p-ee-l* – a facial treatment in which one or more chemicals are applied to remove several layers of sun-damaged skin, leaving fresh skin with a more even surface and colour. It may also stimulate new *collagen* production to improve texture. Superficial peels may be performed by a *beauty therapist* or nurse, but deep peels must be performed by a dermatologist (a doctor who specialises in skin diseases and conditions) or surgeon.

Chemotherapy – *kee-moh-th-e-rap-ee* – a treatment used for some types of cancer and some non-cancerous conditions. It is a *contraindication* for most beauty treatments and the client must seek GP approval first.

Cheque – *ch-e-k* – an order written on a standard printed form, instructing a bank to pay money from the specified account to the person or organisation specified.

33

Chilblain – *ch-il-b-lay-n* – a small area of itchy, red skin most common on the toes. It is a painful, abnormal reaction of the small *blood vessels* in the skin when exposed to cold temperatures. It occurs when *constriction* of the blood vessels in response to cold is followed by rapid rewarming of the skin. This causes leakage into the *tissues* as the blood vessels do not respond quickly enough.

Chloasma – *klo-as-ma* – a blotchy, brown colouring in the skin that develops slowly and may fade in time. It is especially common in women between the ages of 20 and 40 and occurs frequently during pregnancy, or as a side effect of the contraceptive pill. It may also occur with sun exposure after applying chemicals such as perfume, scented toiletries, aftershave or deodorant to the skin. This is called a phototoxic reaction and is due to *ultraviolet radiation* being absorbed by the chemical substance on the skin.

Cholesterol – *kol-es-t-rol* – a white substance found in the *tissues* of the body and in certain foods such as animal fats, egg yolks and oil. It is linked to heart disease and *atherosclerosis* as it collects on the walls of the *arteries* and interferes with the flow of blood.

Chromosome – *kr-oh-mo-so-m* – a single *molecule* of *DNA*.

Chyme – *k-eye-m* – a liquid substance found in the stomach, consisting of partially digested food.

Cilia – *sil-ee-a* – tiny, hair-like projections on the surface of some cells. Cilia line the nose and passages in the *respiratory system* and remove foreign bodies (objects coming from outside the body) before they reach the lungs. Also the name for eyelashes.

Circulatory system – *ser-q-lay-tor-ee sis-t-m* – the transport system for blood around the body, consisting of the heart and *blood vessels*. The blood vessels carry blood containing food, *hormones*, *metabolic waste* and gases (oxygen and carbon dioxide) to and from cells. The circulatory system has three distinct parts: the pulmonary circulation (the movement of blood to the lungs and back to the heart); the systemic circulation (the movement of blood to the rest of the body and back to the heart) and the coronary circulation (the circulation within the heart). (See the diagram on page 199.) Also known as the *cardiovascular system*.

Clapping – *klap-ing* – a *percussion* massage technique performed with the hands in a slightly cupped position. The therapist *flexes* and *extends* the wrists while dropping the hands rapidly but lightly onto the client's body. The hands spring back quickly, creating a hollow sound. Clapping is stimulating and increases warmth in the *tissues*. Also known as cupping.

Clavicle – *k-lav-i-kl* – the collar bone. (See the diagram on page 195.)

Cleanser – *k-lens-r* – a product used on the skin to remove makeup, surface oil, pollutants and dead skin cells. Cleansers are made for different *skin types*, usually from a mixture of oil and water with an *emulsifier* added to hold the mix together. They may also have additional ingredients such as *essential oils* to provide fragrance and therapeutic effects.

The percentage of oil to water will determine the consistency, which can range from a liquid to a cream. The ideal cleanser will clean the skin without upsetting the skin's *pH* balance.

Cleansing cream – *k-lens-ing k-ree-m* – a water in oil *emulsion*, varying in consistency from a light mousse to a thick cream. Most suitable for *dry*, *mature* and *dehydrated skin* types, as it has a higher oil to water content. It is easy to apply without dragging and leaves the skin feeling smoother.

Cleansing lotion – *klens-ing low-sh-on* – a liquid *cleanser* with added alcohol, often used with water and ideal for *oily* and *congested skins*.

Cleansing milk – *klens-ing mill-k* – an oil in water *emulsion* with up to 90% water, making it into a free-flowing, milky cleanser ideal for younger skins, as it feels cool and grease-free. Sometimes contains a cosmetic detergent to control *bacteria* and oil production.

Cleansing wipes – *klens-ing w-eye-p-s* – pre-moistened (continued) pads for cleansing, impregnated with makeup remover. They are used for home care and are suitable for all skin types.

Clear wrap – *kl-ee-r rap* – a thin, transparent plastic film used to protect or insulate eyelashes during an **eyelash perm** or on the hands and feet after applying cream and before placing them in **thermal mittens** or bootees. Also known as cling film.

Client – *kl-eye-en-t* – a person (or group of people) who pays for professional services.

Client commitment – *kl-eye-en-t kom-it-men-t* – the agreement of the client to a particular course of action, e.g. booking a course of treatments or buying a product.

Client preparation – *kl-eye-en-t prep-a-ray-shon* – a procedure carried out before treatment, to ensure client comfort and that the **treatment** will be carried out effectively. The preparation required will depend on the treatment given. For example, preparation for a **facial** includes providing a gown, slippers and towels to cover the client and maintain modesty, removing jewellery, adjusting the facial couch to ensure client comfort, protecting the client's hair and checking for **contraindications**.

Closing a sale – *kl-oh-sing a say-l* – the stage of selling a product or service when the client or customer commits to buying.

Club hair – *kl-ub her* – a hair in the **catagen** stage of hair growth which has become detached from the dermal **papilla** and has lost its

Client groups – *kl-eye-en-t gr-oop-s* – refers to client diversity. The ethnic group classification used by the Commission for Racial Equality (CRE) is: White, Mixed, Black, Asian and Chinese.

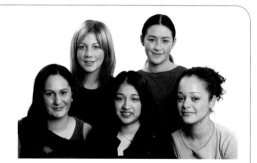

Some ethnic skin types

bulb-like root, forming a club-shaped base. (See the diagram on page 191.)

Coagulate – *koh-ag-you-lay-t* – to change from a liquid to a soft, jelly-like mass, as in normal blood clotting.

Code of conduct – *k-oh-d of kon-duk-t* – a set of business *ethics* that explain the values, responsibilities, obligations and ethical aims of an organisation and the way in which it functions. It provides guidance to employees or members about the right course of action in order to maintain professional standards. Also known as a code of ethics.

Code of practice – *k-oh-d of pr-ak-tis* – the correct actions, methods or processes to be followed in an organisation in order to comply with the rules of the organisation.

Collagen – *kol-a-jen* – the main *protein* of *connective tissue*. It has great strength and is the main component of *cartilage*, ligaments (tissue joining bones together at a joint), *tendons*, bone and teeth. It also provides strength to *blood vessels*. Together with soft *keratin*, it is responsible for skin strength and *elasticity*. The breakdown of collagen leads to the wrinkles that accompany ageing. Collagen is a good water-binding agent (helps the skin to retain moisture).

Collagen therapy – *kol-a-jen th-er-rap-ee* – the injection of *collagen* into the skin to fill out lines, wrinkles and pitted *scars*.

Colour therapy – *kul-or th-e-rap-ee* – the use of colour to balance emotional and spiritual health, dating back to Egyptian times. Colour may be *(continued)*

Cold sore – *k-old s-or* – an eruption on the face, usually around the mouth or nose area, which may accompany a cold or be triggered by *stress* or sun exposure. It is characterised by redness and small *vesicles*. See also *herpes simplex*.

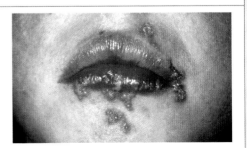

A cold sore

37

used in the decoration of a room, the fabrics used or with adjustable lighting.

Combination skin – *kom-bin-ay-shon s-k-in* – a skin that has characteristics of more than one *skin type*: *dry*, *oily*, *normal*, *mature* or *sensitive skin*. The most common combination is an oily 'T' zone across the forehead and down the centre panel of the face over the nose and chin, with drier areas on the cheeks and neck.

Comedo – *kom-e-d-oh* (plural **comedones** – *kom-e-d-ohn-s*) – a plug of *sebum* and *keratin* blocking the duct (channel) of a *sebaceous gland*. Sebum is trapped in the mouth of the *follicle* and turns black when exposed to oxygen. Also known as a blackhead.

Comedogenic – *kom-e-doh-jen-ik* – tending to block pores, cause *comedones* or aggravate *acne*.

Commission – *kom-i-sh-on* – a percentage of the selling price of a product or treatment paid to the therapist for each sale made.

Commitment – *kom-mit-men-t* – a pledge, promise or obligation.

Communication – *ko-m-you-nik-ay-shon* – the exchange of thoughts, messages or information through speech, behaviour, writing or signals.

Compact bone – *kom-pak-t b-oh-n* – the outer, dense (thick and solid) layer that forms the shaft of the long bones.

Competence – *kom-p-ten-ss* – ability to form a task well, possession of the required skill, knowledge or qualification.

Complaint – *kom-play-n-t* – an expression of displeasure about behaviour, a service, treatment or product.

Complete – *kom-p-lee-t* – finished, ended or concluded.

Compound follicle – *kom-p-ow-n-d fol-ik-l* – see *pili multigemini*.

Computer – *kom-p-you-t-er* – a programmable electronic device that works at high speed and assembles, stores and processes information. It usually contains a central processing unit and memory, together with a display screen, keyboard, printer and mouse.

Concealer – *kon-see-l-er* – a *makeup* product used to hide blemishes, dark shadows and other marks on the skin.

Conductor – *kon-duk-t-or* – a substance or material that allows electricity or heat to flow along it.

Confidentiality – *kon-fi-den-sh-ee-al-it-ee* – privacy. Confidentiality means protecting all information about a client and not disclosing it to anybody else. Client confidentiality is an important aspect of the beauty business as it instils confidence in the client and demonstrates professionalism.

Congenital – *kon-jen-it-al* – describes something present at birth.

Congested skin – *kon-jest-ed sk-in* – occurs when the *pores* in the skin become blocked so that the *sebum* does not flow freely. This causes a slightly bumpy feel to the skin as the sebum

blockages become hard and *epidermal tissue* forms over the *follicle* openings. This skin type is often accompanied by *milia* and *comedones*. It may be caused by inadequate cleansing, using skin care products that block the pores or by humidity, as this prevents sweat evaporating easily from the surface of the skin.

Conjunctivitis – *kon-jun-k-tiv-eye-tis* – *inflammation* of the transparent *membrane* (conjunctiva) that lines the inner surface of the eyelid and covers the eyeball. Also known as pink eye.

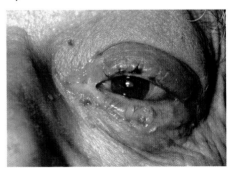
Conjunctivitis

Connective tissue – *kon-ek-tiv ti-shoo* – special structures of cells that support, bind or separate other *tissues* and organs. Connective tissue consists of a base substance made *(continued)* up of salts, water, *protein* and *carbohydrate*, combined with *collagen* for support and *elastin* fibres to provide *elasticity*. It contains specialist cells, including *macrophages* to fight infection, *plasma* cells that produce *antibodies* and *mast cells* that produce *histamine*.

Constriction – *kon-strik-shon* – the act of narrowing or making smaller.

Consult – *kon-sul-t* – to seek advice or information from a professional person.

Consultation – *kon-sul-tay-shon* – a conversation between a client and a therapist to discuss the client's requirements and the objectives of the *treatment*. A detailed consultation is required at the first visit to record personal and medical information to ensure the client receives the most appropriate treatment. *Contraindications* may be identified and **modifications to treatment** agreed if necessary.

Consumer – *kon-s-you-mer* – a person who makes use of services or buys goods.

Contamination – *kon-tam-in-ay-shon* – the presence of *infection*.

Continuing professional development – *con-tin-you-in-g pro-fe-sh-on-l de-vel-op-men-t* – constant improvement of skills and knowledge in order to make progress in a profession.

Contour cosmetics – *kon-tor kos-met-iks* – **blushers**, **highlighters** and **shaders** used to **enhance** and accentuate good features and minimise bad ones. They come in the same formulations as **foundations**: liquid tint, cream, **gel** and pressed and loose powder.

Contouring – *kon-tor-in-g* – making or shaping an outline, e.g. shading underneath the cheekbone with a contour powder to accentuate this feature.

Contra-action – *kon-tra-ak-shon* – an adverse effect on the skin or body during or after a **treatment**.

Contract – *kon-trak-t* – an agreement between two or more people that is legally binding and enforceable by law. A contract is made when an offer made by one person is accepted by another.

Contraction – *kon-trak-shon* – the change in a muscle when it becomes shortened and thickened during normal movement, physical or passive exercise or in reaction to an electrical stimulus.

Contraindication – *kon-tra-in-di-kay-shon* – any reason to prevent or adapt *treatment* or refer to a qualified person for permission to treat. Contraindications may be temporary, specific or general.

Cool wax – *koo-l w-a-ks* – See *warm wax*.

Cooperation – *k-oh-op-er-ay-shon* – working or acting with others for a common goal.

Corn – *k-or-n* – a localised (in one place) area of thickened skin. Caused by friction or pressure stimulating the cells of the *epidermis* (called *keratinocytes*) to increase in number. This results in a thicker *stratum corneum*. Corns are most commonly found on the toes and feet.

Corrugations – *ko-roo-gay-shon-s* – grooves or ridges in the *nail plate*.

Corrugator – *ko-roo-gay-t-or* – a facial *muscle* situated at the corner of each eyebrow which draws the eyebrows downwards and together. (See the diagram on page 192.)

Cortex – *kor-tek-s* – the outer layer of an organ or the outer section of a hair. (See the diagram on page 191.)

Corticosteroid – *kor-tic-oh-ste-roy-d* – a *steroid* that is produced in the adrenal *cortex* (see *adrenal gland*), including *cortisol* and *aldosterone*.

Cortisol – *kor-t-i-sol* – a hormone produced by the adrenal cortex (see adrenal gland). It is involved in glucose metabolism, regulation of blood pressure, insulin release, suppressing the immune system and in response to inflammation. It has been called 'the stress hormone' because it is secreted in high levels during the body's 'fight or flight' response to stress. Small increases of cortisol provide a quick burst of energy, *(continued)* increase memory function and immunity, lower sensitivity to pain and help maintain *homeostasis*.

COSHH (Control of Substances Hazardous to Health) – *ko-sh* – regulations that set out the legal guidelines a business must follow to ensure that hazardous substances are stored, used, handled and disposed of safely.

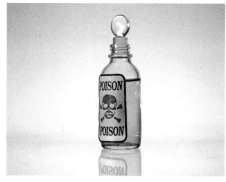

COSHH regulations require hazardous substances to be clearly labelled

Cosmeceuticals – *kos-m-s-you-tik-al-s* – products applied directly to the skin that bring together cosmetics and pharmaceuticals. They combine cosmetic ingredients with ingredients that affect biological functioning to improve the health and appearance of the skin. These products have often been developed by dermatologists (doctors specialising in skin

disorders) and usually contain ingredients such as vitamins, herbs, oils and botanical (from plants) extracts. The manufacturers are not allowed to claim that they penetrate beyond the surface layers of the skin or have any medical effects.

Cosmetic camouflage – *kos-met-ik kam-er-fl-ar-j* – makeup products and techniques used to hide, disguise or correct imperfections in the skin.

Cosmetics – *kos-met-iks* – products used to preserve or restore beauty.

Cost effective – *kos-t ee-fek-tiv* – giving good value for money, or producing a good profit in relation to the outlay.

Counterfeit – *kow-n-ter-fit* – an imitation made fraudulently or deceptively to seem genuine.

Cranium – *kr-ay-nee-um* – the part of the *skull* that provides a protective covering for the brain, composed of several bones fixed together at immovable *joints*. (See the diagram on page 196.)

Cream – *k-ree-m* – a cleansing or moisturising cosmetic with a thick consistency.

Create – *k-ree-ay-t* – to produce from personal ideas and artistic or imaginative effort.

Credit – *kr-ed-it* – an agreement in which someone receives goods or services and pays for them later or in instalments. *Also* a sum of money owed to a person. *Also* a book-keeping term to describe an entry of payment received.

Credit card – *kr-ed-it kar-d* – a card that allows an individual to make purchases using borrowed money. It is only issued when the individual has proved that they have a satisfactory credit rating (i.e. they can be trusted to pay back the money).

Crêpey skin – *kr-ay-pee s-k-in* – lined and wrinkled skin caused by the natural ageing process, sun damage, rapid weight loss, illness or poor skin *elasticity*.

Cross-infection – *kr-oss in-fek-shon* – the spread of disease from one person to another through poor *hygiene* practices.

Cryptosporidium – *krip-t-oh-spo-rid-ee-um* – a *parasite* that is a common cause of the water-borne disease cryptosporidiosis, which causes diarrhoea. The disease may be caught by swallowing infected water from swimming pools, hot tubs, spas, jacuzzis, fountains or lakes.

Cuboid – *q-boy-d* – one of the seven *tarsal* bones in the foot.

Cultural awareness – *kul-t-yor-ral a-wer-ness* – knowledge and understanding of the behaviour, beliefs and characteristics of a particular social, ethnic or age group.

Cuneiform bones – *q-ni-for-m b-oh-n-s* – three bones in the foot, located between the *navicular* and the first three *metatarsal* bones. (See the diagram on page 197.)

Currency – *ku-ren-see* – money in any form used in exchange for goods and services.

Current assets – *ku-ren-t ass-e-t-s* – cash owned by a business and other possessions which can easily be sold and converted into cash.

Current trends – *ku-ren-t t-r-end-s* – the most recent fashion, style or designs.

Cushing's syndrome – *k-ush-in-g-z sin-d-r-oh-m* – a condition of the *endocrine system* caused by an over-*secretion* of *cortisol* from the *adrenal glands*. The most common cause is Cushing's disease, in which the *pituitary gland* produces too much *adrenocorticotrophic hormone* (ACTH). This stimulates the adrenal glands to produce cortisol. Other causes are *tumour* of the pituitary or adrenal gland, or long-term use of corticosteroids (a type of *steroid*). Symptoms may include a round face, obesity of the *abdomen*, thin arms and legs, thin skin that is easily bruised, increased urine production, excess facial hair, no *menstruation*, impotence, *acne*, general weakness, thirst, backache and headache.

Cutaneous – *q-t-ay-nee-us* – relating to the skin.

Cuticle – *q-tik-l* – the outer layer of cells in the hair. *Also epidermal tissue* above the *matrix* of the nail at the base of the *nail plate*.

Cuticle cream – *q-tik-l c-ree-m* – a mixture of fats and waxes used to replace lost oil and moisture and soften and nourish the *cuticle*, allowing it to be pushed back with ease.

Cuticle knife – *q-tik-l n-eye-f* – an implement used in *manicure* and *pedicure* to remove traces of *cuticle* from the *nail plate*.

Cuticle nippers – *q-tik-l nip-er-s* – an implement used in *manicure* and *pedicure* to trim torn or ragged *cuticles*.

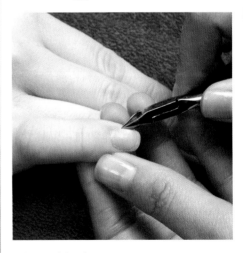

Using cuticle nippers

Cuticle remover – *q-tik-l re-moo-v-r* – a lotion applied to the *cuticle* to aid in its removal. This product may have an irritating and drying effect on the skin and nail because it is highly *alkaline*, so it should be applied in moderation and removed quickly after use.

Cuticle work – *q-tik-l wer-k* – treatment of the *cuticles* of the nail, including moisturising, pushing back and trimming. This *enhances* the appearance of the *nail plate*, discourages the formation of *hangnails* and ensures a clean surface on which to apply nail enamel.

Cutting – *ku-tin-g* – to trim or shorten with scissors, clippers or knife.

Cyst – *sis-t-s* – a small cavity that forms a closed sac (pouch) containing fluid, semi-solid matter or air. Cysts can occur anywhere in the body and may be single or multiple. Some common cysts include sebaceous cysts (in the skin and filled with *keratin*), ovarian cysts (fluid-filled cysts in the ovary), ganglions (fluid-filled cysts connected to a joint) and popliteal cysts (behind the knee).

Cytoplasm – *s-eye-toe-plas-m* – the jelly-like substance in a *cell* that maintains the cell's shape. It is situated between the *cell membrane* and the *nucleus*. It holds all the organelles (structures within the cell with special functions) of the cell outside the nucleus and stores chemicals that are involved in vital metabolic reactions. (See the diagram on page 188.)

Dappen dish – *da-p-n di-sh* – a small, flat-bottomed dish used to decant (pour from one container to another) small amounts of product during the application of false nail *extensions*. Ideally it should have a lid to prevent evaporation of volatile (evaporate rapidly) liquids. Using a dappen dish avoids contamination of products and reduces wastage by using only the required amount of product.

Data – *day-ta* – facts, statistics or other information collected for analysis or to make decisions.

Data protection – *day-ta pro-tek-shon* – measures taken to ensure the safety of *data* held. A business must comply with the Data Protection Act 1998, which regulates how personal information is used and provides protection from misuse of personal details.

Day spa – *d-ay s-p-ar* – a *spa* that provides therapeutic treatments that last for any amount of time from an hour to a full day. Might be situated in a hotel, department store, health club or on the high street.

Debit card – *deb-it k-ar-d* – a payment method that is an alternative to cash or a cheque. It allows payment to be withdrawn immediately from the cardholder's bank account if the account holds sufficient funds.

Decongestant – *dee-kon-jest-ant* – a substance that reduces congestion (a build-up of blood or *tissue fluid* in an organ or vessel (channel) or a build-up of *sebum*, dead skin cells and *bacteria* in the *hair follicle*) (see *congested skin*).

Deep vein thrombosis (DVT) – *dee-p vay-n th-rom-b-oh-sis* – a blood clot that develops in a deep vein, usually in the lower leg. It may cause pain and swelling of the calf muscle. A potential complication of this condition is pulmonary embolism (a blockage in the pulmonary *artery* – see *pulmonary circulation*), when a piece of the clot breaks off and travels to the lungs. DVT may be caused by a damaged vein or if the flow of blood slows down or stops. There are many risk factors, including heredity, immobility (e.g. on long-haul flights), obesity, age, recent surgery, the contraceptive pill, hormone replacement therapy and treatment for other circulation or heart problems.

Defect – dee-fek-t – an imperfection that may cause inadequacy or failure.

Dehydrated skin – dee-h-eye-dr-ay-ted sk-in – skin lacking moisture. This can happen to all *skin types*. It results in areas of flaky skin and tightness, a dull complexion and makeup application may be streaky. There are several causes: exposure to wind, extreme cold or heat, central heating or air conditioning, harsh products that strip the skin of moisture, shaving, medication and illness or a diet high in salt.

Deltoid – del-toy-d – a triangular *muscle* that covers the shoulder, the action of which raises the arm away from the side of the body.

Demonstrate – dem-on-st-ray-t – to describe, explain or illustrate by using practical examples or experiments.

Demonstration – dem-on-st-ray-shon – an illustration or explanation using practical examples or experiments. Can be used to teach a practical skill or to promote a product, treatment or service.

Dendrites – den-dry-t – branches that extend from the main body of a *neuron* (nerve cell) and receive nerve impulses (signals).

Deoxygenated blood – dee-ox-ij-en-ay-ted b-l-ud – blood that is low in oxgen. (See the diagram on page 198.)

Depilation – dep-il-ay-shon – temporary removal of unwanted hair using *tweezers*, *depilatory creams*, wax, *abrasives*, *sugaring* or mechanical *epilators*.

Depilatory cream – dep-il-at-or-ee kr-ee-m – a product used to temporarily remove unwanted hair from the body. It contains an *alkaline* chemical such as calcium thioglycolate, which dissolves the *protein* structure of the hair. It is also available as a *gel*, foam or roll-on.

Depressor labii – d-pres-or lab-ee-eye – facial *muscle* beneath the lower lip, which pulls *(continued)*

47

the lip down and to one side. (See the diagram on page 192.)

Dermal cord – *der-m-l k-or-d* – a string of cells connecting the *hair follicle* to the *dermal papilla*, supplying blood in the *catagen* and *telogen* stages of the hair growth cycle. It is from these cells that a new follicle will eventually form. (See the diagram on page 190.)

Dermal papilla – *der-m-l pa-pill-a (plural* **papillae** – *der-m-l pa-pill-eye)* – a projection of the *papillary layer* of the dermis containing *blood vessels*, nerve endings or the blood supply that provides nourishment to the *hair follicle*. (See the diagram on page 190.)

Dermatitis – *der-mat-eye-tis* – see *eczema*.

Dermatosis papulosa nigra – *der-mat-t-oh-sis pap-you-loh-sa ni-g-ra* – a harmless skin condition seen mostly on *black skin*. It is characterised by multiple, small, darker *papules* (bumps) on the face, neck, chest and back. It is more common in older people.

Dermis – *d-er-mis* – the second of the three major layers of the skin. It is a layer of dense *connective tissue* beneath the *epidermis* and is composed of three types of tissue: *collagen*, *elastin* and reticular fibres (which form a supporting mesh). The dermis has two layers: the superficial *papillary layer* and the deep reticular layer. The dermis also contains many specialised structures: *hair follicles* with *arrector pili muscles* that cause the hairs to stand on end; *sebaceous glands* that produce *sebum* to lubricate the skin and hair; *sudoriferous glands* to help cool the body and excrete (remove from the body) waste; *blood vessels*; and *sensory nerves*. (See the diagram on page 189.)

Design – *dee-z-eye-n* – to plan and create in an artistic and skilful manner. *Also* a drawing or sketch.

Desincrustation – *de-sin-kr-us-t-ay-shon* – a deep cleansing treatment using the effects of a *galvanic current* to soften the skin and remove surface oil and skin blockages. It is performed on the negative pole and has the effects of increasing circulation, stimulating nerve endings, softening the skin, creating an *alkaline* effect on the surface of the skin and attracting fluid to the area.

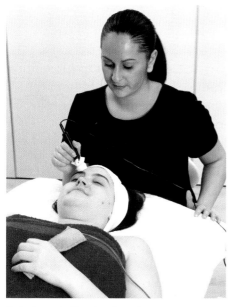

A desincrustation treatment

Desincrustation fluid – *de-sin-kr-us-t-ay-shon fl-oo-id* – a dilute (weak) *alkaline* solution used to deep cleanse and remove excess *sebum* from the skin in a galvanic treatment (see *galvanic unit*).

Desquamation – *des-kwa-may-shon* – the natural process of shedding dead skin cells from the top layer of the *epidermis*, the *stratum corneum*.

Destination spa – *des-tin-ay-shon sp-ar* – a specialist establishment for certain *market niches*, providing an environment and therapies that achieve specific results, such as *lifestyle* enhancement, health benefits or self-improvement. This type of *spa* may also provide outdoor adventure activities, medical treatments, nutritional advice or complementary therapies.

Detoxification – *dee-toks-if-ik-ay-shon* – the use of specific treatments to cleanse the body of impurities and *toxins* that have accumulated.

Diabetes mellitus – *d-eye-a-bee-t-ees mel-it-us* – a lifelong disease characterised by high levels of *glucose* in the blood. The cause is either not enough *insulin* produced by the *pancreas* to regulate blood sugar or resistance to insulin, or sometimes both. Type 1 diabetes is also called insulin-dependent diabetes, and is usually diagnosed in childhood. In this type, the body makes little or no insulin. Type 2 is the most common form of diabetes. It usually occurs gradually in adulthood. In this type, the pancreas does not produce enough insulin to keep *(continued)* 49 blood sugar levels normal. Clients who suffer from diabetes may have delicate skin that bruises easily and poor circulation, contributing to slower skin healing. Some treatments may be *contraindicated* and the therapist should adapt or modify treatment depending how severe the condition is and any side effects that are present.

Diaphragm – d-eye-a-fr-am – a dome-shaped *muscle* that separates the thoracic (in the chest) and abdominal (in the *abdomen*) cavities. It extends across the bottom of the rib cage and is an important muscle in breathing. The diaphragm contracts and flattens when *inhaling*, enlarging the thoracic cavity and allowing air to be drawn into the lungs. When *exhaling*, the diaphragm relaxes, reducing the size of the thoracic cavity and forcing air out of the lungs.

Diastolic pressure – d-eye-as-tol-ik pre-sh-or – the minimum pressure in the *arteries* during relaxation and *dilation* of the heart, the second number recorded in a blood pressure reading.

Diathermy – d-eye-a-th-er-m-ee – the production of heat in a part of the body, using a high-frequency current.

Diet – d-eye-et – all the foods that a person regularly eats. *Also* a particular selection of food chosen to improve a person's physical condition or to prevent or treat a disease. *Also* to limit the amount of food eaten in order to lose weight.

Differentiation – dif-er-en-see-ay-shon – the specialisation of different types of cells to carry out specific functions in the body. *Also* the differences that make one business better than the competition.

Diffusion – di-f-you-sh-on – the movement of particles in liquids or gases from a high concentration on one side of a thin *membrane* to a low concentration on the other side.

Digastric – d-eye-gas-trik – a deep *muscle* under the chin attached to the *mandible*, *temporal bone* and *hyoid bone*. It helps in moving the tongue and swallowing. (See the table on page 194.)

Digestion – *d-eye-jes-t-y-on* – the process by which food is broken down into *molecules* small enough to be absorbed by the cells and used by the body for growth, energy, maintenance and repair. It is the second of four stages: *ingestion*, digestion, *absorption* and *excretion*.

Digestive system – *d-eye-jes-tiv sis-t-m* – a series of organs and *glands* in the body that prepare food for use by the cells. It consists mainly of a long, twisting tube that runs from the mouth, where the food enters the body, to the anus, where waste products from the digestive process are eliminated from the body. It consists of the mouth, salivary glands, *oesophagus*, stomach, liver, *pancreas*, large intestine, small intestine, rectum and anus. The functions are movement, *secretion*, *digestion*, *absorption* and *elimination*.

Digits – *di-j-it-s* – fingers or toes.

Dilated capillaries – *d-eye-lay-ted ka-pil-a-r-ee-s* – *capillaries* that have been enlarged due to some stimulation (an action that causes a response). They fail to return to their original size because their walls lose their *elasticity*.

Dilation – *d-eye-lay-shon* – enlargement or widening. Occurs in the *blood vessels* when body temperature rises, allowing blood to be transported to the skin and so heat is lost, helping the body to cool down.

Dilator naris – *d-eye-lay-t-er n-ar-is* – part of the *nasalis* muscle situated at the sides of the nostrils, the action of which is to dilate (expand) the nostrils. (See the diagram on page 192.)

Direct current (DC) – *d-eye-rek-t ku-rent* – a constant electric current flowing in one direction, produced using batteries. Also a rectified, smoothed *alternating current* which has been converted from alternating to direct.

Disability discrimination – *dis-ab-il-i-tee dis-krim-in-ay-shon* – to treat a person with a physical or mental disability differently from others.

Disciplinary procedure – *dis-i-plin-a-ree pr-oh-see-d-your* – action or process to investigate a reported breach of *(continued)* discipline within an organisation.

Discount – *dis-k-ow-n-t* – a reduced price offer for goods or services.

Discrepancies – *dis-krep-n-see-s* – differences or inconsistencies.

Discrimination – *dis-krim-in-ay-shon* – making a distinction in favour of or against a person, based on the group to which that person belongs rather than on individual merit.

Discussion – *dis-kus-shon* – an informal debate or exchange of views between two or more people.

Disease – *dis-ee-s* – a condition affecting the body as a result of *infection*, *genetic* defect or a stressful environment, which is characterised by an identifiable group of signs or symptoms. Presence of a disease will normally be a *contraindication* to treatment or require *modification to treatment*.

Disinfectant – *dis-in-fek-t-ant* – a chemical substance that completely destroys *bacteria*.

Disorder – *dis-or-der* – an ailment affecting the function of the mind or body.

Dispute – *dis-p-you-t* – a quarrel, argument or disagreement.

Distal – *dis-t-l* – furthest away from the point of origin.

Disulphide bond – *d-eye-sul-f-eye-d bon-d* – a cross-linking chemical bond (an interaction between atoms and molecules that provides stability) containing two atoms of sulphur, which hold together and stabilise two *protein* chains (a group of proteins bonded together like the links in a chain). Hair proteins are held together by disulphide bonds, which are broken down and then reformed during the process of *eyelash perming*.

Diuretic – *d-eye-or-et-ik* – a substance or drug that increases the volume of urine excreted (removed from the body) by the kidneys.

DNA (Deoxyribonucleic acid) – a *molecule* that is present in the *nucleus* of all living cells. It contains the *genetic* instructions for the development and function of living things. The DNA segments that carry this information are called *genes*. Human DNA is often referred to as the blueprint of the human body.

Dorsiflexion – *dor-see-flek-shon* – raising the foot by pointing the toes upwards.

Dosha – *do-sh-er* – a Sanskrit word used to describe the three types of *metabolism* according to Ayurvedic medicine: Vata, Pitta and Kapha. Each dosha is a combination of two elements: Vata is space and air, Pitta is fire and water, Kapha is water and earth. See also *Ayurveda*.

Dry flotation – *dr-eye fl-oh-t-ay-shon* – a relaxing therapy in which the body floats without getting wet and which is combined with other treatments. The body is covered in oils, creams or mud for a therapeutic purpose and is then wrapped in a plastic blanket that is filled with water. The surrounding warm water allows the products to penetrate more deeply or work more effectively.

Dry skin – *dr-eye s-k-in* – a *skin type* that results from a lack of moisture in the *stratum corneum*. The characteristics include thin *epidermis*, pale colour, patchy skin, rough texture, lack of oil, underactive *sebaceous glands* and a tight feeling after washing. It may be caused by the environment, inherited factors, using harsh products, age, medication, an underactive *thyroid gland* or skin conditions such as *eczema* or *psoriasis*.

Duodenum – *due-oh-dee-num* – the upper part of the small intestine leading from the stomach to the *jejunum*.

Duties – *d-you-tee-s* – actions and tasks that someone has to carry out for moral or legal reasons.

Dysmenorrhoea – *dis-men-or-ee-a* – painful menstruation.

Ear lobe – *ee-er low-b* – the outer part of the ear that can be seen. Also known as pinna or auricle.

Eccrine glands – *ek-r-ee-n gl-and-s* – **sweat glands** with ducts (channels) opening directly onto the surface of the skin. They are linked to the **sympathetic nervous system** and help to regulate body temperature. They are found all over the body, but more abundantly on the soles of the feet, palms of the hands and forehead. They produce **sweat**, which is composed mainly of water and salts.

Ecospa – *ee-ko s-par* – a type of **spa** that has been established in a natural or protected area and that has been designed and is run in an environmentally friendly manner. Ecospas use organic and indigenous (found locally) ingredients and educate clients about environmental issues.

Ectomorph – *ek-toe-mor-f* – a lean and angular body shape, thin with narrow hips and shoulders and very little body fat or muscle.

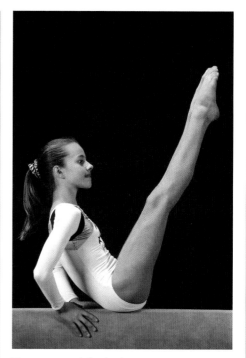

The ectomorph body shape

Eczema – *ek-z-ma* – **inflammation** of the skin, which may cause dryness, flaking, reddening of the skin and itching. Itchy **blisters** may develop, which if scratched may burst and crust over. Eczema is caused by many things but most commonly it is an **allergy** to a substance such as detergent, soap, perfume, cosmetics, oils, chemicals and some foods. Also known as dermatitis.

Efferent – *e-f-e-ren-t* – describes a vessel (channel) or nerve that carries a substance or impulse away from an organ or body part to another part of the body. For example, efferent *lymph vessels* carry *lymph* away from a *lymph node*.

Effleurage – *ef-le-rar-j* – a soothing, stroking movement in *massage*, which is used to begin, finish and link other massage movements. It is performed with the flat of the hand using long, flowing strokes. Slightly more pressure is applied with the first stroke, towards the heart, and lighter pressure in the return movement.

Eggshell nails – *egg-sh-el n-ay-l-z* – thin, pale and fragile nails curved at the *free edge*, caused by internal *disease*, poor *diet*, medication or disorders of the *nervous system*.

Elasticity – *el-as-tis-it-ee* – the ability of *tissue* to return to its original shape after *contraction* (shortening) or *extension* (stretching or lengthening).

Elastin – *el-as-tin* – a protein similar to *collagen*. It is the main component of elastic fibres in the skin, providing the skin with *elasticity*.

Electric current – *e-lek-tr-ik ku-ren-t* – a flow of *electrons* along a circuit, measured in *amperes*. It is used in *electrotherapy* beauty treatments to achieve deeper effects than are possible using manual techniques. An electric current may be used to produce: heat (e.g. a *sauna*, *steam bath*, spa pool, *infrared* lamp, *paraffin wax*); sound waves (e.g. from *audiosonic* massage equipment); chemical effects (e.g. in a galvanic treatment – see *galvanic unit*); light rays (e.g. from infrared and ultraviolet lamps) or movement (e.g. in a *faradic treatment*).

Electrical epilation – *e-lek-tr-ik-l e-pil-ay-shon* – the complete removal of hair from the root by destruction of the *dermal papilla* by means of *diathermy* using a high-frequency current, *electrolysis* using a direct *galvanic current* or *thermolysis*. These methods may be used in combination – called *blend epilation*.

Electrical facial – *e-lek-tr-ik-l fay-sh-l* – a specialised manual *facial* treatment that incorporates one or more pieces of *(continued)* electrical equipment to increase the effects and the *benefits* to the client. Equipment may include *microcurrent*, *high-frequency current* (direct or indirect), *iontophoresis*, *desincrustation*, a *faradic unit*, *vacuum suction*, *microdermabrasion*, *intense pulsed light* or *laser*.

Electrical muscle stimulation (EMS) – *e-lek-tr-ik-l mus-el stim-you-lay-shon* – see *faradic treatment*.

Electrode – *e-lek-tr-oh-d* – an *applicator* or *conductor* used to apply an *electric current* to the body.

Electrolysis – *e-lek-tr-ol-i-sis* – the popular term used to describe the permanent removal of unwanted hair using a *galvanic current*, or a blend of galvanic and *thermolysis* methods. It is the destruction of living *tissue*, especially of *hair roots*, by means of a current applied with a needle *electrode*, more commonly called a probe.

Electrolyte – *e-lek-tro-l-eye-t* – any compound that separates into *ions* when dissolved in water and is able to conduct (carry) electricity.

Electromagnetic spectrum – *e-lek-tr-oh-mag-net-ik sp-ek-tr-um* – the range of all possible electromagnetic (referring to magnetism produced by electric charge in motion) *radiation*. In order of frequency from lowest to highest, this includes radio waves, microwaves, *infrared* radiation, visible light, *ultraviolet radiation*, x-rays and gamma rays.

Electron – *e-lek-tr-on* – a particle with a negative charge that circles the *nucleus* of an *atom*.

Electronic authorisation – *e-lek-tr-on-ik or-th-or-eye-say-shon* – permission or approval received for payment after entering a personal identification number (PIN) into an electronic terminal.

Electronic cash register – *e-lek-tr-on-ik k-ash rej-is-ter* – an electronic till point that records payment, calculates bills, issues receipts and provides a safe place to store cash and other valuables.

Electronic mail – *e-lek-tr-on-ik may-l* – an instant message passed from one computer to another by typing the message and sending it through a computer or mobile phone, WiFi (Wireless Fidelity) device or PDA (Personal Digital Assistant – a small, hand-held computer used as a personal organiser). Commonly known as email.

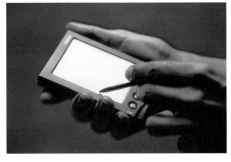

A PDA

Electrotherapy – *e-lek-tr-oh-th-er-ap-ee* – the use of mechanical or electrical equipment in facial and body *treatments* for a therapeutic purpose. Mechanical methods include: vibratory (capable of producing vibration), *massage*, microdermabrasion and *vacuum suction*. Electrical equipment includes: *high-frequency*, *galvanic*, *faradic* and *microcurrent* units.

Elimination – *e-lim-in-ay-shon* – the act of removing or getting rid of something. *Also* the act of *excretion* (getting rid of waste products or foreign substances from the body).

Emergency – *ee-mer-jen-see* – a sudden, unexpected occurrence requiring immediate, urgent action.

Emerging trends – *ee-mer-jin-g tr-en-d-s* – styles or fashions that are currently developing gradually.

Emery board – *em-er-ee b-or-d* – a small, stiff strip of cardboard or paper coated with powdered emery (a very hard mineral) and used in *manicure* and *pedicure* to shorten or file the nails.

Emollient – *em-oh-lee-ent* – a soothing, softening substance applied to the skin, which also helps to prevent water loss.

Emulsify – *em-ul-s-if-eye* – to combine two liquids that do not normally mix easily, such as oil and water.

Emulsion – *em-ul-shon* – a mixture of oil, water and an added ingredient called a 'surfactant', which helps the oil and water to mix. Used to massage the body and moisturise the skin.

Endermologie – *en-der-moll-o-jee* – a specialised electrical massage treatment designed to treat **cellulite**.

Endocrine gland – *end-o-cry-n gl-and* – a ductless (without a channel leading from it) organ that secretes (releases) **hormones** into the blood. Endocrine glands are an important part of the **endocrine system**.

Endocrine system – *end-o-cry-n sis-t-m* – a system of **glands** that works together with the **nervous system** to control the activity of internal organs, **cells** and body functions. It helps to regulate mood, growth and development, **tissue** function, sexual function, reproductive processes and **metabolism**. Endocrine glands include the **hypothalamus**, **pineal gland**, **pituitary gland**, **thyroid gland**, **parathyroid glands**, **thymus gland**, **adrenal glands**, **pancreas**, **ovaries** and **testes**. (See the diagram on page 200.)

Endometrium – *end-oh-mee-tree-um* – the inner lining of the **uterus**.

Endomorph – *end-oh-mor-f* – a round body shape with narrow shoulders, which may have wide hips and a high proportion of body fat.

Endorphin – *end-or-fin* – a chemical compound that occurs naturally in the brain, acts as a painkiller and is responsible for feelings of pleasure.

Enfleurage – *on-fl-er-ar-j* – an early method used to extract **essential oils** from flowers. The flowers are pressed into vegetable or animal fat and the essential oils seep into the fat, which is eventually washed with alcohol to separate the essence from the fat. The alcohol is then left to evaporate, leaving the essential oil.

Enhance – *en-han-s* – to improve or add to.

Enquiry – *en-kw-eye-r-ee-s* – a question or query in order to find out information.

Ensure – *en-sh-or* – to make sure or certain.

Environmental conditions – *en-v-eye-ron-men-t-l kon-dish-on-s* – the state of the setting, surroundings or area. For example, to provide the right environmental conditions for a body massage treatment, the room would require warmth, subdued lighting, an adjustable couch, a private changing area and a quiet atmosphere, whereas a manicure would require a brightly lit room, a manicure table and a supportive chair for the client to sit on.

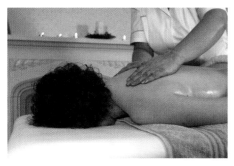

The environmental conditions must be appropriate for the treatment

Enzymes – *en-z-eye-m-s* – *protein molecules* produced by living *cells* that act as catalysts (substances that cause or speed up a chemical reaction). Used in *cosmetics*, enzymes help in *exfoliation* of the skin and improve texture.

Eosinophils – *ee-o-sin-o-fil-s* – *white blood cells* that destroy *parasites* and play a role in *allergic* reactions.

Epidermal tissue – *ep-ee-der-mal tis-you* – *tissue* forming the outermost layer of the skin.

Epidermis – *ep-ee-der-mis* – the outermost layer of skin, above the *dermis*. It contains no blood vessels and consists of five layers: the *stratum germinativum*, *stratum spinosum*, *stratum granulosum*, *stratum lucidum* and *stratum corneum*.

Epilate – *e-pill-ay-t* – to remove hair from the body by means of physical, chemical or electrical means.

Epilation needle – *e-pil-ay-shon nee-d-l* – a fine probe, the same diameter as a hair, used in electrical epilation. It is inserted into the *hair follicle* to direct the current flow. There are different types, including: a flexible two-piece; a more rigid one-piece; gold (which is suitable for *sensitive skin* as it is *hypoallergenic*, inserts more smoothly into the follicle and conducts (carries) the current more effectively); stainless steel; and insulated (which is suitable for the *flash technique* and for sensitive skin). The needles are available in sizes from 2 to 6 and size 10 for advanced *(continued)* techniques. The smaller the number the thinner the needle.

Epilator – *e-pil-ay-tor* – a mechanical device for temporary hair removal. Epilators have an electric rubber roller or coiled spring that catches the hair and pulls it out by the root. They have different speeds and strengths and some have an optional shaving unit for skin areas too sensitive for the *plucking* action.

Epilepsy – *e-pil-ep-see* – a condition that causes the sufferer to have recurring attacks known as seizures. These happen when there is an abnormal electrical discharge in the brain, disturbing its normal function. Bright lights may be a trigger. The condition is controlled by medication but is a *contraindication* to many beauty treatments, for which the client must seek GP approval first.

Epiphora – *e-pi-for-a* – see *watery eyes*.

Epithelial tissue – *e-pith-ee-lee-al tis-you* – specialised *tissue* that covers all external and internal surfaces of the body. It is made up of *cells* closely packed together in one or more layers.

The epithelial tissue covering internal surfaces is called endothelium. Epithelial tissue is separated from the tissue underneath by a thin sheet of *connective tissue* called the basement *membrane*. This provides structural support and binds the epithelial tissue to neighbouring structures. Simple epithelium is one cell thick and stratified epithelium is two or more cells thick.

Eponychium – *ep-o-nik-ee-um* – *cuticle* or skin at the base of the *nail plate*. *Also* the name given to *epidermal tissue* over the developing fingernail of a foetus (unborn baby).

Equal opportunities – *ee-k-wol op-or-t-you-nit-ee-s* – the provision of an acceptable social environment, in which every person has the same chances in life and will not be discriminated against, regardless of age, gender, ethnic group, marital status or sexual orientation.

Erector spinae – *ee-rek-tor sp-eye-n-eye* – deep *muscles* located along the spine. They are the strongest muscles in the back and are arranged in three vertical columns: spinalis (*medial* column), longissimus (intermediate column) and iliocostalis (**lateral** column). They keep the body in an erect (straight) position when sitting or standing. When **flexed**, they straighten the spine and bend it backwards.

Erythema – *e-ri-th-ee-ma* – reddening of the skin due to **dilation** of the **capillaries**. This occurs in some people as a response to manual or mechanical **treatment**, after exposure to **ultraviolet radiation**, or due to illness or high fever.

Erythrocyte – *e-ri-th-r-oh-s-eye-t* – a red blood cell that contains **haemoglobin** to carry oxygen from the lungs to the body's **tissues**.

Essential oils – *ee-sen-t-sh-al oy-l-s* – the fragrant essences of plants, herbs, flowers, leaves, berries, fruits, bark, resin, seeds, wood, roots, grasses, etc. They are extracted for therapeutic use and for their perfume. They are classified as top, middle and base notes. Top notes are light and fresh, middle notes provide the heart of a fragrance and base notes are rich and heavy in aroma.

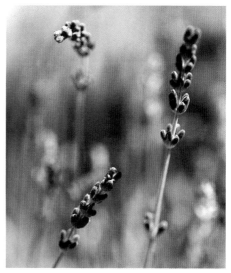

Lavender is one of the most versatile essential oils

Establish – *es-tab-li-sh* – to start up, install or settle into position. *Also* to prove to be valid or true.

Ethics – *e-th-iks* – a system of moral principles or rules of conduct recognised by a particular group, profession or organisation. All professions have their own particular **code of conduct**, which states the standard of behaviour required by their members and which is recorded in a professional code of ethics.

Ethmoid – e-th-moy-d – a small bone in the *cranium*, filled with air spaces. It forms part of the nasal cavity (the air passage behind the nose) and the eye sockets.

Evaluate – ee-val-you-ay-t – to estimate, judge, calculate or determine the importance or value of something.

Evening primrose oil – ee-v-nin-g prim-r-oh-s oy-l – a *carrier oil* used in *aromatherapy*. It is fine-textured and has *anti-inflammatory* and *emollient* effects, making it a superb moisturiser. It can be used to improve *eczema*, *psoriasis*, premenstrual syndrome and rheumatoid *arthritis* (a chronic and disabling *autoimmune disease* affecting the *joints*). It is obtained from the seeds of the oil of the evening primrose flower and has been used medicinally for centuries.

Exchange – ex-ch-ayn-j – to change one item for another.

Excretion – ex-k-ree-shon – the process of eliminating (getting rid of) the waste products of

metabolism from the body as water, *urine* and *carbon dioxide*.

Excretory system – ex-kree-tor-ee sis-t-m – a major system in the body that controls the volume of body fluids and what they contain, as well as eliminating (getting rid of) body waste.

Exfoliant – ex-f-oh-lee-ant – a cosmetic product or ingredient used to remove dead skin cells. It may be chemical or mechanical. Also known as an exfoliator.

Exfoliation – ex-f-oh-lee-ay-shon – the manual or mechanical method of removing dead skin cells from the *epidermis* using a technique such as loofah scrub, dry brushing, *salt rub*, *enzyme* masks, *abrasive* scrub or microdermabrasion.

Exhalation – ex-h-a-lay-shon – breathing out, pushing out air from the lungs.

Exhale – ex-hay-l – to breathe out.

Exocrine gland – ex-o-cry-n gl-and – an organ that secretes (releases) substances through a duct (a channel through which fluid is conveyed).

Expression – *ex-pr-e-shon* – a method for extracting **essential oils** from citrus fruits. (Also known as the cold press method.) The essential oil is squeezed from the rind or peel of the fruit. *Also* a look or reaction on the face that shows feelings and emotions.

Extend – *ex-ten-d* – to increase the length, or to straighten and stretch out to the full length.

Extensibility – *ex-ten-si-bil-it-ee* – the ability of **tissue** to be stretched when pulled.

Extension – *ex-ten-shon* – an increase in the angle between two bones. *Also* an addition to an existing part, e.g. the addition of a false eyelash or nail.

Eye cream – *eye k-r-ee-m* – a specially formulated product for the eye area, used to nourish the skin and prevent lines and wrinkles forming.

Eye gel – *eye jel* – a cooling and soothing product, usually made from gentle plant and herb extracts such as **chamomile** and cornflower, used on the eye area to revitalise tired eyes, reduce the effects of puffiness and firm the skin.

Eye makeup remover – *eye may-kup re-moo-v-er* – a special **cleanser** formulated for the delicate eye area, made from **gels**, oils, creams or lotions. It is gentle in effect and helps to remove stubborn eye **makeup**, in particular waterproof **mascara**. Special eye makeup remover pads are also available for clients to use at home.

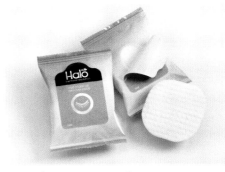

Eye makeup remover pads

Eye shadow – *eye sh-add-oh* – a **cosmetic** used to add colour and dimension to the eyes. It comes as powder, cream, **gel**, watercolours, pencils or minerals.

Eyebrow – *eye-br-ow* – the bony ridge extending over *(continued)* the eye and covered by an arch of short hairs that provides a frame for the eye.

Eyebrow shaping – *eye b-r-ow sh-ay-pin-g* – a procedure carried out in a salon to *enhance* the eyes and provide character to the face. Manual or automatic *tweezers* are used to pluck individual hairs from beneath the brow to make the eyes look larger and allow eye *makeup* to be applied more effectively. *Threading* or *waxing* may also be used if the client prefers.

Eyelash – *eye l-ash* – short hairs fringing the edge of the eyelid. False eyelashes and *extensions* may be applied to *enhance* the natural lashes or they may be permed or tinted to improve the appearance.

Eyelash and eyebrow tinting – *eye-l-ash and eye-brow tin-t-ing* – a salon procedure to darken or change the colour of the eyebrows and eyelashes. A small amount of *tint* is mixed with peroxide to a smooth paste, applied to the hairs and left for the required time before removal. It is ideal for people who are sensitive to *mascara* and cannot wear *makeup*, for contact lens

wearers and swimmers, for people going on holiday, to emphasise colour intensity for light hair colour and for those with no time to apply makeup.

Eyelash perming – *eye l-ash p-er-min-g* – a temporary method of curling the upper lashes through 'chemical re-formation'. The hair's chemical bonds (*disulphide bonds*) are broken down and then re-formed in a new shape. This treatment is provided for clients with short, straight lashes to give definition to the eye, for clients who do not like wearing *mascara* or cannot because of a job, a sport or sensitivity to eye *makeup*, and also for photographs or special occasions. The lashes are curled over small rods, a perm solution is applied to soften the hair, which then moulds to the shape of the rod, and finally a fixing solution or *neutraliser* is applied to fix the curl in place.

Eyeliner – *eye-l-eye-ner* – a *cosmetic* for the eyes, applied close to the lashes in a thin line to accentuate the eyes. Colour can be chosen to blend with the eyelashes or eye shadow.

Face mask – f-ay-s m-as-k – a preparation applied to the skin as part of a *facial* to reinforce cleansing of the skin. The mask may be ready-made and contained in a tube or pot, or a combination of ingredients that are mixed together to form a paste or *gel*, to suit the client's *skin type*. Other effects, depending on ingredients, are nourishing, hydrating (moisturising), soothing, refining, peeling, desquamating (shedding of dead skin cells) or thermal (heating). Masks may be setting and become hard in a short time or non-setting and remain flexible until removed. Specialised face masks may be made from a material infused (soaked) with an active ingredient such as *collagen*, or come in the form of wax, *gel* or oil. Biological masks may be made from fruit, plants or herbs – the trace elements (very small amounts of chemicals) in the ingredients increase cellular activity in the *basal layer* of the *epidermis*.

Face powder – f-ay-s pow-der – a fine-milled powder used to set *makeup*, provide a base on the eyelid for shadow, *blend* harsh lines and for use throughout the day when the skin looks shiny.

Available in many different shades and textures.

Facial – f-ay-sh-l – a therapeutic beauty *treatment* using manual techniques, designed to improve all skin conditions. It includes a thorough cleanse, *exfoliation*, massage, application of one or more *face masks*, hydration (moisturising) and protection. The effects achieved are cleansing, exfoliating, toning, hydrating, protecting, relaxing and maintaining a healthy skin.

Facial massage – f-ay-sh-l mass-ar-j – a relaxing part of the *facial* performed after the skin has been cleansed, exfoliated and any other preparatory treatments have been carried out. Massage oil or cream is used to allow a smooth flowing treatment, together with the massage techniques of *effleurage*, *petrissage*, *percussion* (continued)

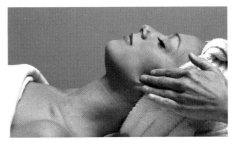

A facial massage

and *vibrations*, using firm but even pressure and a steady rhythm. This helps to promote relaxation, remove tension, improve skin texture and stimulate circulation.

Facial nerve – *f-ay-sh-l n-er-v* – mainly a *motor nerve* of facial *expression*, it also has a small sensory (to do with the senses) part which carries impulses (signals) from the taste buds and salivary *glands*. It is divided into five branches: temporal, zygomatic, buccal, mandibular and cervical.

Facial scrub – *f-ay-sh-l s-kr-ub* – a cleansing product containing an *abrasive* ingredient such as crushed nut kernel, oatmeal, synthetic (not natural) micro beads or salt used to exfoliate the skin and provide a smooth surface.

Facial steaming – *f-ay-sh-l s-tee-min-g* – a heat treatment during a *facial*. Gently heated water is used to produce a light vapour that is directed onto the skin. It is used to preheat, cleanse or hydrate the skin, open the *pores*, soften skin blockages and increase *desquamation*. The heat

applied will increase circulation and the flow of *lymph*, bringing nourishment to the area and removing waste products through perspiration (*sweat*).

Faeces – *f-ee-see-s* – semi-solid material containing undigested food, *bacteria* and fluid that is produced in the large intestine and eliminated (removed) from the body.

Faradic current – *fa-ra-dik ku-rent* – a short-duration (time), interrupted or surged (coming in waves), low-frequency *direct current*. It is a safe current used in body and facial therapy to improve *muscle tone* and condition through passive exercise.

Faradic treatment – *fa-ra-dik tr-ee-t-men-t* – a form of passive muscle exercise treatment (the individual is inactive; the exercise is performed by the *electric current* when applied to the body) using a *faradic unit*. It is a popular salon treatment for body toning and firming, using a *faradic current* to produce muscle *contractions*. The current is applied to the body via *electrodes* placed on a muscle or muscle group and this stimulates the muscles, helping to tighten, lift and firm body contours. Smaller electrodes are used on the face, allowing the therapist to target individual muscles or the *facial nerve*, which stimulates several muscles at once, improving conditions such as a double chin, drooping eyelids, deep *nasolabial folds* or a dropped jaw line. Also known as passive muscle exercise, electrical muscle stimulation (EMS) or neuromuscular electrical stimulation (NMES).

Faradic unit – *fa-ra-dik you-nit* – the machine used to provide passive *muscle* exercise treatment for face and body, using a *faradic current*.

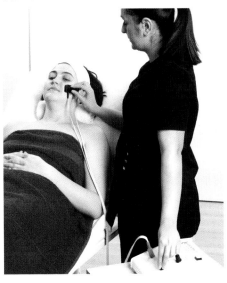

A facial faradic treatment

Fascia – *fa-see-a* – a sheet or band of fibrous (consisting of fibres) *tissue*.

Fax machine – *f-aks ma-sh-ee-n* – a piece of electronic equipment that sends and receives printed messages and images over a telephone line by converting them to and from electronic signals.

Features – *fee-t-y-or-s* – the qualities, characteristics and prominent or distinctive aspects of a product or *treatment*. Knowing the features is an important part of selling, as it allows the therapist to describe products with knowledge, instilling confidence in the client and thus contributing to making the sale.

Femur – *fee-m-r* – the upper leg or thigh bone. (See the diagram on page 195.)

Fibreglass wrap – *f-eye-b-gl-ass rap* – a strengthening layer used when creating a nail *extension*. It is durable (long-lasting) and strong, thin but loosely woven, to allow *adhesive* to penetrate easily. Also known as a fibreglass overlay.

Fibril – *fib-ril* – a thin, threadlike strand which makes up a **cell** or larger structure. Fibrils make up the contractile (capable of **contraction**) part of **skeletal muscle**.

Fibrin – *fib-r-in* – a **protein** that is necessary in helping blood to clot.

Fibroblasts – *f-eye-br-oh-bl-as-t-s* – **cells** found in **connective tissue** that secrete (release) **elastin** and **collagen protein** fibres.

Fibula – *fib-you-la* – the outer and thinner bone of the two bones that form the lower leg. It extends from the knee to the ankle.

Filing – *f-eye-lin-g* – a method in **manicure** and **pedicure** using an **emery board** to reduce the length of or shape the **nail plate** or to smooth sharp or rough edges.

Fire escape – *f-eye-er es-k-ay-p* – a stairway on the outside wall of a building. It provides an emergency exit in the event of fire or other emergency when the stairways inside the building are inaccessible.

Fire exit – *f-eye-er ex-it* – a special door to be used in emergencies such as fire. It is an outward-opening door with an easy-to-open crash bar and exit signs leading to it. It is normally located at the bottom of a flight of stairs or in a hallway to allow fast evacuation of a building in case of fire. It can also be a main doorway in or out of the building. Also known as emergency exit.

Fire extinguisher – *f-eye-er ex-tin-gw-i-sh-r* – a portable, manually operated container filled with **carbon dioxide**, foam, dry powder or water that can be sprayed in a steady stream to put out a small fire. Each type has a coloured panel indicating the contents: black (carbon dioxide); cream (foam); blue (powder); and red (water).

First aid – *fer-s-t ay-d* – emergency help or treatment given to an injured or ill person while waiting for professional medical care.

Fixed assets – *fi-ks-d ass-e-t-s* – the long-term resources of a business, e.g. buildings, equipment and furniture.

Fixed cost – *fi-ks-d k-os-t* – a business cost that does not change, e.g. monthly rent.

Flammable – *fl-am-a-b-l* – easily set on fire and capable of burning rapidly.

Flash technique – *f-l-ash tek-nee-k* – a method of **electrical epilation** used in short-wave **diathermy**, in which a high-intensity current is used for a very short space of time.

Flatstones – *f-lat st-oh-n-s* – tiny, flat holograms (three-dimensional pictures or images), solid and hollow shapes used as a decorative item in nail art. They are flexible to use, allowing ease of application to the nail.

Flex – *f-l-ek-s* – to bend a part of the body at a **joint**.

Flexible – *fl-ek-s-i-b-l* – easily moved, capable of being bent without breaking. *Also* able to change easily to adapt to a situation.

Flexion – *fl-ek-sh-on* – reduction in the angle between two bones, as in bending.

Flotation – *fl-oh-t-ay-shon* – the act, process or condition of floating in water. It is a name given to a water therapy in which the client lies in a tank filled with water treated with a high concentration of Epsom salts (natural salts obtained from mineral spring water used to reduce inflammation). The high density of the solution allows the body to float naturally and effortlessly. The benefits are relief from pain, relaxation, an increased sense of well-being and restoration of **homeostasis**.

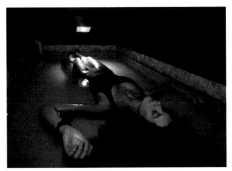

A flotation tank

Foam bath – *f-oh-m b-a-th* – a form of **hydrotherapy** in which a bath is filled with water and heated to a temperature of 38–43°C and a foaming *(continued)*

69

essence is added. An air compressor is switched on to aerate (cause air to circulate through) the water and form bubbles. The bubbles provide insulation (prevent heat loss) for the client sitting in the bath, creating and maintaining heat to relax the client, ease muscular tension, stimulate the skin and induce perspiration (sweating).

Foiling – *f-oy-lin-g* – a technique used in nail art design: the application of metallic, coloured and patterned foil to the nail to create a pattern.

Follicle – *fol-ik-l* – a small cavity (space), sac (pouch) or *gland* in the skin, generally having a secretory (discharging a substance) function. Examples are *hair follicles* (see the diagram on page 191), *ovarian* follicles, *lymph* follicles and *thyroid* follicles.

Follicle stimulating hormone (FSH) – *fol-ik-l st-im-you-lay-tin-g h-or-m-oh-n* – a *hormone* secreted (released) by the *anterior pituitary gland* that promotes the formation of ova (eggs) in the female and sperm in the male.

Folliculitis – *fol-lik-you-l-eye-t-is* – *inflammation* of one or more *hair follicles* resulting in a tender, red spot often with a *pustule* on the surface. It may be caused by: *bacterial* infection (*Staphylococcus aureus*) or spa pool folliculitis (*Pseudomonas aeruginosa*) from water without enough chlorine; yeast infection (*Pityrosporum ovale*), causing an itchy, *acne*-like condition affecting the upper trunk of a young adult; or *fungi* (*Tinea capitis*), causing *ringworm* of the scalp.

Foot spa – *f-u-t s-par* – a small bubble bath for the feet. This is an ideal accompaniment to a *pedicure* for cleansing and relaxation. It provides a soothing treatment with jet massage to remove *stress* and soothe tired feet. It may be a small, free-standing piece of equipment or combined into a special pedicure couch.

Foramen magnum – *for-ar-men mag-num* – a large opening in the lower part of the occipital bone (situated at the base of the skull at the back), through which the spinal cord (part of the *central nervous system*) passes.

Foundation – f-ow-n-day-sh-on – a *cosmetic* that creates a smooth, even-toned finish to the skin. Foundations come in many different forms: mousse, cream (water in oil), liquid (oil in water), compact, *gel* and fine spray mist.

Fragrance – fr-ay-gr-an-s – a volatile (evaporates rapidly) oil or blend of oils that provide a pleasant aroma in products. Can be botanical (from plants) or synthetic (manufactured).

Franchise – fr-an-ch-eye-s – a licence given by a successful company to an individual or group to market its products or services in a specific area and to make use of the company's name, reputation and expertise.

Franchisee – fr-an-ch-eye-s-ee – a person or company to whom a *franchise* is granted. This allows them to use a well-established business idea for a certain cost.

Franchisor – fr-an-ch-eye-s-or – a person or company who grants a *franchise* to another person, giving them the right to use their name and business idea.

Fraud – f-r-or-d – deceit and trickery, an unlawful act for profit or gain.

Freckles – fr-ek-l-s – small, brown, areas of skin that develop in sun-exposed areas and are most common on fair skin types, particularly those with red hair who have an inherited tendency for freckles. Freckles may be present at birth. They are caused by increased *melanin* production and become darker when exposed to the sun. Also known as ephelides. See also *lentigo*.

Free edge – fr-ee ed-j – the *distal* (furthest away from the body) end of the *nail plate* which can be filed and shaped. (See the diagram on page 190.)

Free radicals – fr-ee rad-ik-l-s – highly reactive chemicals that attack *molecules* by capturing *electrons* and change their chemical structure. Environmental factors such as pollution, *ultraviolet radiation* (UVA rays), smoking and pesticides may cause free radical damage. If production of free radicals becomes excessive, damage occurs and this accumulates with age.

French manicure – *fr-en-ch man-ik-your* – a particular method of applying enamel to the nails. The first application is a pink, translucent (semi-transparent) base – a colour close to the colour of the **nail bed** for a natural look. Then a white tip is applied to the free edge, using an opaque (not clear) enamel, and finally a top coat is applied to form a seal.

Frequency – *fr-ee-qw-en-see* – the number of waves, vibrations or cycles per second.

Frictions – *fr-ik-shon-s* – small, deep *massage* manipulations using pressure to break down adhesions (fibrous bands of *tissue*), loosen *scar* tissue and increase *joint* mobility. Frictions are performed with the thumb or fingertips in circles or across the area being massaged.

Frigidarium – *fr-i-jid-er-ee-um* – the final room in the original Roman baths. A cold room with a refreshing and invigorating cold plunge pool.

Frontalis – *fr-un-t-ar-lis* – the *muscle* of the forehead covering the frontal bone of the skull. It raises the eyebrows and wrinkles the forehead horizontally. (See the diagram on page 192.)

Frosted polish – *fr-os-ted po-li-sh* – nail enamel with a shiny, shimmery effect. Also called **pearlised polish**.

Frothing – *fr-o-th-in-g* – the escape of hydrogen and chloride gases from the **hair follicle** as a result of treatment with *galvanic current* or *blend epilation* (see *electrical epilation*).

Fruit acids – *fr-oo-t as-id-s* – organic acids derived from fruit and used in skin *exfoliation*. Available as cream, lotion or a gentle peel treatment, they include grapes, apples, pineapple, citrus fruits, papaya and blackberries. They may be incorporated into home care products or in higher concentrations in a professional treatment.

Fuller's earth – *ful-er-s er-th* – a type of clay that has been finely milled to produce a useful ingredient in *face masks*. It has excellent absorbent properties, making it ideal for use on an *oily skin*, for its deep cleansing and drying effects. It is highly stimulating and slightly bleaching in effect.

Fungus – *fun-gus* (plural **fungi** – *fun-g-ee*) – a type of simple organism including yeast, moulds and mushrooms. Certain types of fungi are responsible for *infections* that may occur anywhere on the body. They usually affect the skin because they live on *keratin*, the *protein* that makes up skin, hair and nails.

Furrows – *fu-r-oh-s* – deep ridges in the nail which may be caused by poor *nutrition*, injury to the *matrix* or illness. Constant rubbing of the cuticle can cause friction in the area of the matrix and deep ridges, which then grow up the *nail plate* until they reach the *free edge*.

Fuse – *f-you-s* – a safety device to protect electrical circuits from excessive amounts of current. If the current is too high, the metal wire in the fuse melts and breaks the circuit.

Gain – *g-ay-n* – to obtain something through personal effort.

Galvanic burn – *gal-van-ik b-er-n* – a chemical burn, caused by a concentration of acids or bases on the skin during galvanic treatment (see *galvanic unit*). The *tissue* damage is deep but concentrated in a tiny area and a black mark on the skin may form as a result. Chemical burns are also caused by substances such as bleach or pool chlorinator.

Galvanic current – *gal-van-ik ku-ren-t* – a constant direct *electric current* used in body and facial therapy to improve skin and body condition and aid in hair removal.

Galvanic unit – *gal-van-ik yoo-nit* – a piece of electrical equipment used to provide galvanic treatment with a constant *direct current* on the negative or positive pole. It is used in two ways on the face: *desincrustation* to deep cleanse an oily or blemished skin and *iontophoresis* to introduce products deep into the skin for a specific purpose such as hydrating, soothing or healing.

When used on the body it helps in the treatment of *cellulite*.

Gamma irradiation – *ga-ma i-ray-dee-ay-sh-on* – a physical means of *sterilisation* or decontamination (destruction of harmful substances). Electromagnetic rays (waves of energy in the *electromagnetic spectrum*) of extremely short wavelength are emitted. These pass through the treated product and disrupt the organic processes that cause contamination. Gamma irradiation is used to sterilise *epilation needles* or probes.

Gaseous exchange – *gas-ee-us x-ch-ay-n-j* – the *exchange* of oxygen and carbon dioxide in the body. This takes place in the lungs by *diffusion* through the *alveoli*.

Gastrocnemius – *gas-tr-ok-nee-me-us* – a powerful *muscle* situated in the back part of the lower leg, beneath the knee and down to the heel. Together with the *soleus* it forms the calf muscle. Its main action is *plantarflexion* of the foot (pointing the foot downwards). It also helps to *flex* the knee *joint*. (See the diagram on page 202.)

Gel – *jel* – a jelly-like material used in cosmetic preparations, which liquefies (changes from a gel to a liquid state) when warmed.

Gel nails – *jel-nay-l-z* – application of a *gel* over a plastic nail tip to produce a natural-looking false nail with a high gloss finish. The gel is set hard by using *ultraviolet* light or spraying with setting gels.

Gender dysphoria – *jen-der dis-for-ee-a* – a condition where a person of one gender identifies strongly with the other gender. They may undergo hormone and surgical treatment to physically change their sex.

Gene – *j-ee-n* – a unit of *genetic* material or *DNA*, inherited from a parent. Genes determine the characteristics of each individual.

Genetic – *j-en-et-ik* – inherited, often occurring within the same family.

Germicide – *jer-miss-eye-d* – an agent that kills germs.

Germinative layer – *jer-min-ay-tiv lay-er* – see *stratum germinativum*.

Gesture – *jest-yer-s* – a movement of the hands or limbs used to help express thoughts or to add emphasis to the spoken word.

Gland – *g-l-and* – an organ of the body that produces a *secretion* such as saliva, *hormones*, mucus, tears, *bile* or *sebum* for release into the blood, into body cavities or onto the body's outer surface.

Glitter – *gl-it-ter* – a product used for nail art design consisting of fine, sparkly dust. It is applied to the nails by dragging or dotting and may also be mixed with acrylic powder, ultraviolet *gel* or nail enamel. Glitter can also be an ingredient in makeup products to add sparkle.

Glomerulus – *gl-o-mer-you-lus* – a mass of tiny *blood vessels* located in the kidney in an area called the Bowman's capsule. It is the main filter of the nephron (the functional unit of the kidney). It is semi-permeable (allowing only certain substances to *(continued)*

75

pass through) – water and soluble substances pass through and are excreted (removed from the body) from the kidneys as urine.

Glucagon – *gl-oo-cag-on* – a *hormone* secreted by the *pancreas* that increases the level of *glucose* in the blood.

Glucocorticoids – *gl-oo-koh-cor-tik-oy-d-s* – a group of *hormones* produced in the adrenal *cortex* (see *adrenal gland*). Their function is to raise the level of blood sugar (*glucose*).

Glucose – *gl-oo-koh-s* – a sugar that occurs in animal *tissues* and fluids and in fruits. It is the main type of sugar circulating in the blood and the main energy source of the body.

Gluteal – *gl-oo-t-ee-al* – relating to the buttocks.

Gluteals – *gl-oo-t-ee-al-s* – three *muscles* (the gluteus maximus, medius and minimus) which together make up the buttocks. Gluteus maximus is the largest and it contributes to the shape of the buttocks. It helps to maintain the body in the erect

(straight) position and rotates and *extends* the hip *joint*. The gluteus medius and minimus help to abduct (see *abduction*) the hip and rotate the thigh.

Glycerin – *g-lis-er-in* – a substance present in all natural fats which helps protect the skin by attracting the right amount of water to maintain the skin's *homeostasis*. Also known as glycerol.

Glycerine – *g-lis-err-ee-n* – a colourless, odourless, sticky and thick, non-toxic liquid with a sweet taste, used as a cleansing ingredient in soap and *face masks*. It is kind to the skin and is also used in facial creams and body lotions as a *moisturiser*.

Glycogen – *gl-eye-ko-jen* – a form of *carbohydrate* that is stored in the body, mainly in the liver and muscle *tissue*. It is quickly converted into *glucose* when it is needed to satisfy the body's energy needs.

Glycolic acid – *gl-eye-kol-ik a-sid* – the most common *alpha hydroxy acid* found in *cosmetic* preparations. It has a small molecular structure (is made of tiny parts) and so penetrates (enters) the skin quickly. It is most suitable for *mature* and *oily skin* or for people with sun-damaged skin or *acne*. Products containing glycolic acid are manufactured in different formulations: *gels*, creams, lotions and serums at varying *pH* levels and concentrations.

Goitre – *g-oy-t-er* – enlargement of the *thyroid gland*.

Golgi tendon organ – *g-ol-g-ee ten-don or-g-n* – a sensory receptor (receives messages from the *nervous system*) organ situated at the junction between a *tendon* and a *skeletal muscle*. It provides information about changes in muscle tension.

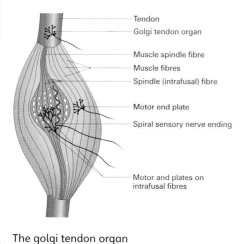

Tendon
Golgi tendon organ

Muscle spindle fibre
Muscle fibres
Spindle (intrafusal) fibre

Motor end plate
Spiral sensory nerve ending

Motor and plates on intrafusal fibres

The golgi tendon organ

Gonads – *go-nad-s* – the sex glands – *ovaries* and *testes*. (See the diagram on page 200.)

Gonadotrophin – *go-nad-o-tr-of-in* – a *hormone* that stimulates the growth and activity of the *gonads*.

Gout – *g-ow-t* – a condition characterised by an excess of uric acid (a byproduct of normal *metabolism*) and urates (salt of uric acid) in the blood. It causes pain and *inflammation* in the *joints* of the feet and hands, in particular the joint of the big toe.

GP referral – *jee-pee r-fer-r-l* – directing someone to a general practitioner (doctor) for help or information.

Granular layer – *gr-an-you-l-ar l-ay-er* – see *stratum granulosum*.

Grapeseed oil – *gr-ay-p-s-ee-d oy-l* – a fine-textured, almost odourless (without smell) *carrier oil* used in *aromatherapy*. It is moisturising and regenerative (renews or restores).

Grievance procedure – *gr-ee-v-an-s pr-oh-see-d-yor* – the action taken to resolve problems if an employee wishes to make a complaint or raise issues with an employer. There is a set of steps known as 'the statutory minimum procedures' that have to be included in order to ensure that everybody is treated the same way in similar circumstances, that issues are dealt with fairly and that procedures comply with current *legislation*.

Guidelines – *g-eye-d-l-eye-n-s* – rules and recommendations for how things should be done or how an employee should carry out their job role.

Gyratory massager – *j-eye-ray-tor-ee mass-ar-j-er* – a machine that provides a mechanical method of *massage*. It has several different *applicator* heads, made from sponge for *effleurage* movements and polyurethane and rubber for *petrissage* movements, all used during treatment to achieve similar effects to manual massage. The applicator head works by vibrating horizontally and vertically, creating movement up and down as well as a rapid movement from side to side.

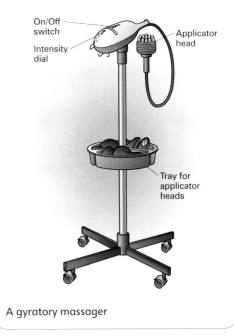

On/Off switch

Intensity dial

Applicator head

Tray for applicator heads

A gyratory massager

Hacking – *ha-king* – a *percussion* movement in *massage* performed across *muscle* fibres with both hands working alternately. The sides of the fingers should strike the area rapidly, producing light, flicking movements.

Haematoma – *hee-ma-toe-ma* – a swelling filled with blood.

Haemoglobin – *hee-mo-glo-bin* – a *protein* that occurs in red blood cells and transports *oxygen* around the body in the blood. It contains iron and provides the red colour of blood.

Haemophilia – *hee-mo-fil-ia* – an inherited blood condition passed from the female to the male, in which an essential blood clotting factor, factor V111, is partly or completely missing. This makes the body less able to control bleeding when injured. The main danger for the sufferer is internal bleeding, into *joints*, soft *tissues* and *muscles*.

Hair bulb – *h-air bu-l-b* – a structure of actively growing *cells*, at the base of the *hair follicle*, which eventually form the hair. The lower part of the bulb is

called the *matrix* – this is where cells are multiplying. In the upper part of the bulb the cells undergo change in growth and development and arrange themselves into six layers. Three inner layers form the hair and three outer layers form the lining of the hair follicle. Special cells called *melanocytes* in the bulb produce *melanin*, the *pigment* that colours the hair. (See the diagram on page 190.)

Hair follicle – *h-air fol-ik-l* – a structure in the *epidermis*, extending into the *dermis*, that contains the *hair root* from which the hair develops. It provides protection for the hair as it grows. It is well supplied with *blood vessels* and the blood supply provides the constant source of nourishment necessary for growth. (See the diagram on page 191.)

Hair germ cells – *h-air j-er-m sel-s* – the *cells* in the skin that start the growth of a new hair.

Hair growth – *h-air gr-oh-th* – the growth rate of hair is *genetically* determined but it may change depending on age and *hormones*. The hair on *(continued)* the head is programmed to grow for years at a time, so that it can grow very long, whereas the hair on the body is programmed to stop growing every couple of months, so that it remains short. Hair growth on the face and body may be defined as **congenital**, topical and systemic. Congenital means present from birth and is determined by inherited **genes**. Abnormal congenital hair growth is a rare condition characterised by **superfluous** hair growth either at birth or later in life. Topical hair growth is a response to stimulation or friction of the **epidermis**, which causes the blood supply to increase and supplies extra nourishment to the **hair follicle**, accelerating hair growth. The hairs in the area grow coarser and deeper, providing protection against further irritation. Systemic hair growth occurs during **puberty**, pregnancy and the **menopause**, when the changes occurring in the body result in a change in the pattern of hair growth. Certain disorders of the **endocrine system** also result in superfluous hair growth, including **Cushing's syndrome**, **adrenogenital syndrome**, **acromegaly** and **polycystic ovarian syndrome**.

Hair root – *h-air r-oo-t* – situated below the surface of the skin and enclosed within the **hair follicle**. The hair root contains the **dermal papilla**, which is fed by the bloodstream and has receptors (special **cells** or **sensory nerve** endings that respond to stimuli) for male **hormones** and **androgens**. Androgens regulate hair growth in the scalp hair.

Hair shaft – *h-air sh-aft* – the hair that can be seen above the scalp, consisting mainly of dead cells that have turned into **keratin** and small amounts of water. It has three layers: the innermost layer or **medulla**, which is only present in large, thick hairs; the middle layer or **cortex**, which provides the hair with **elasticity** and curl; and the outer layer or **cuticle**, which is made up of six to ten overlapping layers of cells and whose main function is to protect the cortex. (See the diagram on page 191.)

Hair types – *h-air t-eye-p-s* – there are three types of hair: *lanugo hair* (which develops on an unborn baby and sheds about four weeks before the baby is born); *vellus hair* (fine, soft hair); and *terminal hair* (which is longer, thicker and coarser than vellus hair). Terminal hair generally has a longer *anagen* phase and its growth is affected by *hormones*, whereas the growth of vellus hair is not. Different ethnic groups have different patterns and types of hair growth. Hair may be further classified as single, compound, curly and corkscrew. Single hair describes one hair growing from one *hair follicle*, while compound hair describes two or more hairs growing from a follicle that has two or more *dermal papillae*. Curly hair has a curved follicle. Corkscrew hair has a distorted follicle.

Half moon – *h-ar-f m-oo-n* – a crescent-shaped, whitish area at the base of the *nail bed* of the finger or toe nail. It is made up of immature nail cells that have not been completely keratinised (see *keratinasation*) and flattened. As these cells move forward to form the *nail plate* they become flat, hard and transparent. (See the diagram on page 190.)

Hallux valgus – *hal-lux val-gus* – see *bunion*.

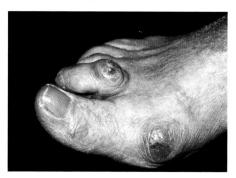

Bunions

Hamstrings – *ham-st-rin-g-s* – a group of three muscles on the *posterior* thigh: the biceps femoris, semimembranosus and semitendinosus. They **extend** the hip and *flex* the knee, playing an important part in everyday activities such as walking, running and jumping. (See the diagram on page 202.)

Hand cream – *h-and kr-ee-m* – an *emollient* or moisturising cream used in *manicure* to massage the hands and arms and replace the natural moisture in the skin and nails. It may also be used in the form of a lotion or *emulsion*.

Hangnail – *h-an-g-n-ay-l* – a common condition in *(continued)* which the *cuticle* around the nail splits. It is caused by dry cuticles or incorrect use of *cuticle nippers*. If left untreated, it may become infected, so it should be carefully removed and the cuticles moisturised to keep them supple and prevent more hangnails developing.

Hard skin remover – *h-ar-d s-k-in re-moo-ver* – an implement such as a pumice stone or file, or a product such as an exfoliating cream or scrub, used in *pedicure* to remove hard skin from the feet.

Hazard – *haz-ar-d* – a possible source of danger.

Hazardous substances – *haz-ar-dus sub-s-tan-ses* – products that pose a risk to health if they are not handled, stored, used and disposed of correctly.

Hazelnut oil – *hay-z-el nut oy-l* – a *carrier oil* used in aromatherapy. It penetrates (enters) the skin quickly and is good for *oily* or *combination skin* or skin that is prone to *acne*. It has toning and tightening effects, encourages regeneration (renewal) of *cells* and strengthens *capillaries*.

Headband – *hed ban-d* – a stretchy band of material, such as towelling or nylon, which is placed around the client's hairline to protect the hair from creams and oils applied to the skin during facial treatment.

Health and safety – *hel-th and say-f-tee* – freedom from disease, illness and from the risk of injury.

Health and Safety Executive (HSE) – *hel-th and say-f-tee x-ec-you-tiv* – the authority that enforces the regulations of the Health and Safety Commission – the body responsible for health and safety legislation in the UK to ensure that risks to people's *health and safety* from activities at work and in many other situations are properly controlled.

Heart – *h-art* – a muscular organ in the body with four chambers, two atria (plural of *atrium*, the upper chamber of the heart) and two *ventricles* (the lower chambers of the heart). It pumps blood received from *veins* into *arteries*, maintaining the flow of blood through the *circulatory system*. The right side of the heart collects *deoxygenated blood* from the veins and pumps it to the lungs. The left side receives *oxygenated* blood from the lungs and pumps it to the *aorta*, which transfers it to the arteries. (See the diagram on page 198.)

Heat treatment – *hee-t tree-t-men-t* – the use of a warm environment or equipment for therapeutic purposes. Several forms of heat treatment are popular in spas and salons to relax or cleanse the body and prepare it for further treatment. Examples are: *sauna*, *steam bath*, *thermal* blanket, *infrared* and *hot stone therapy*.

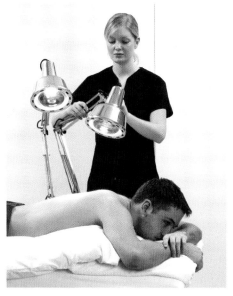

Infrared heat treatment

Heat rash – *hee-t r-a-sh* – an eruption on the skin, accompanied by itching and prickling sensations, usually as a response to a form of heat, including *ultraviolet radiation*.

Herpes simplex – *her-pee-s sim-pl-ex* – an inflammatory skin disease caused by a *virus* and characterised by the formation of clusters of small, fluid-filled *vesicles* and redness. Type 1 is responsible for causing oral herpes (*cold sore*) and Type 2 genital herpes.

Hertz – *her-t-z* – a unit of *frequency* used to measure electrical cycles per second – one Hertz is one cycle per second.

High-frequency current – *h-eye fr-ee-kwe-n-see kur-en-t* – an *alternating current* that oscillates (changes direction) at very high speed. It may be applied directly or indirectly to the body and face.

High-frequency unit – *h-eye fr-ee-kwe-n-see you-nit* – a machine used to provide direct and indirect *high-frequency current*. The direct method is used to deep cleanse an oily, congested, blemished or *(continued)* dull skin; the indirect method is used with a facial massage to allow hydrating and nourishing products to penetrate deeper and faster into the skin.

Highlighter – *h-eye lie-t-er* – used to camouflage (conceal) deep lines such as **nasolabial folds** or to draw attention to good points such as cheekbones and eyes.

Hirsutism – *her-s-you-tiz-um* – excessive hair growth in a woman, following a male growth pattern (e.g. around the chin, on the chest and thighs). It is often **genetic** in origin but may also be caused by increased **androgen** production, age, drugs, **polycystic ovarian syndrome**, pregnancy or a **tumour** on the **adrenal gland**.

Histamine – *his-t-a-m-ee-n* – a substance released from certain cells, in particular **mast cells**, into the body in response to injury or irritation. Histamine causes **dilation** of blood **capillaries**, which can make the skin appear red and feel warm. It also makes the capillaries more **permeable**, allowing fluid to escape into the **tissues**.

HIV (Human Immunodeficiency Virus) – the **virus** that causes **AIDS**.

Hives – *h-eye-v-s* – a lumpy, itchy **rash** that resembles nettle rash, with pale, tiny **vesicles** surrounded by red, inflamed skin. It is a common **allergic** reaction resulting from the release of **histamine** that is often accompanied by swelling of the **tissues**, eyes, ears or lips. Also known as **urticaria** or nettle rash.

Holocrine gland – *hol-o-cry-n gl-and* – a type of **exocrine gland** (a **gland** that secretes externally through a duct, e.g. a sweat gland). Holocrine **secretions** are produced within a cell and the **cell membrane** then ruptures (breaks), releasing the contents. The **sebaceous gland** in the skin is a holocrine gland.

Home care advice – *h-oh-m ker ad-v-eye-s* – opinions and professional recommendations provided by the therapist to the client about products to use at home and how to use them, to ensure the **benefits** achieved through **treatment** are maintained.

Homeostasis – *ho-me-o-st-as-is* – the internal (inside) regulation of the body, so that all the body's systems remain balanced and stable, despite variations in external (outside) influences.

Homeostatic mechanisms – *ho-me-o-st-at-ik mek-an-is-m-s* – the processes by which the body maintains *homeostasis* (remains stable and balanced). These are: osmoregulation (maintaining the amount of water and mineral salts at a constant level); thermoregulation (maintaining body temperature at a constant 36°C); and regulation of blood sugar levels.

Hoof stick – *h-oo-f st-ik* – a wooden or plastic *manicure* or *pedicure* tool with a rubber tip, used to gently push back the *cuticle* without causing damage.

Hormone – *h-or-m-own* – a chemical secreted (released) by the *endocrine glands* that has a *physiological effect* on target cells in the body, causing them to alter their activity.

Hormone replacement therapy (HRT) – *h-or-m-own ree-play-s-men-t th-e-rap-ee* – the use of artificial *oestrogen* and *progesterone* to treat symptoms of the *menopause* such as hot flushes, vaginal dryness and night sweats and also to slow the development of *osteoporosis*.

Horny layer – *h-or-nee lay-er* – see *stratum corneum*.

Hot stone therapy – *hot-st-oh-n th-e-rap-ee* – a relaxing *massage* treatment using heated stones.

Hot wax – *hot w-a-ks* – a form of depilatory (removes hair) *wax* heated to a higher temperature than *warm wax*: approximately 50–55°C. It is made from a mixture of waxes, *resins* and soothing agents and is effective in removal of strong, coarse hair, particularly on the underarm and the bikini line. It is liquid on application, flexible while cooling and brittle when cold.

Humectant – *h-you-mek-tan-t* – a substance that attracts water *molecules* from the surrounding environment, used in some *moisturisers*.

Humidity – *h-you-mid-it-ee* – the amount of water *(continued)*

85

vapour in the air. Higher humidity makes it feel hotter because it reduces the effectiveness of the sweating mechanism to reduce body temperature by preventing the evaporation (disappearance) of *sweat* from the skin.

Hyaluronic acid – *hy-al-yor-on-ik a-sid* – a natural component of *connective tissue*, the function of which is to cushion and lubricate. In skin tissue it is a jelly-like substance that fills the space between *collagen* and *elastin* fibres, providing a transport mechanism to take essential *nutrients* from the bloodstream to living skin *cells*. It hydrates the skin by holding water. Synthetic (artificial) forms have been manufactured for use as dermal (skin) fillers to rejuvenate the appearance and reduce depressions in the skin due to *scars*, injury or lines.

Hydrogen peroxide – *h-eye-dr-o-jen pe-rox-eye-d* – an oxidising agent (a substance that provides oxygen) used to activate eyelash tint. When the liquid hydrogen peroxide is mixed with the tint, oxygen is released. This attaches itself to the *molecules* in the tint, causing the colour molecules to increase in size. When applied to the hair the tint penetrates the *cuticle* and the colour molecules continue to grow in size, allowing the tint to change the colour of the hair.

Hydrophilic – *h-eye-dr-oh-fil-ik* – readily absorbing moisture.

Hydrotherapy – *h-eye-dr-oh-th-e-rap-ee* – the use of water to provide a relaxing and therapeutic treatment and relief from aches and pains. It is one of the oldest forms of medical *treatment*, now used extensively in *spas*. It is carried out at various temperatures and includes *sauna*, *steam bath*, showers, baths, plunge pools, underwater jet massage, *body wraps* and many other treatments.

Hygiene – *h-eye-j-ee-n* – conditions and practices that promote and preserve health by maintaining cleanliness and preventing *cross-infection*.

Hygrometer – *h-eye-grom-e-ter* – an instrument for measuring the water vapour content in the atmosphere.

Hyoid bone – *h-eye-oy-d b-oh-n* – a small bone in the throat, which helps to support the tongue and is an attachment point for several muscles that raise the larynx (upper throat containing the vocal cords) during speech and swallowing.

Hyper- – *h-eye-p-er* – a prefix (beginning part of a word) meaning excessive or abnormally increased.

Hyperaemia – *h-eye-per-ee-m-ee-a* – an instant reddening of the skin due to *dilation* of the *capillaries* in response to an external (outside) stimulus.

Hyperhidrosis – *h-eye-per-h-eye-dr-oh-sis* – excessive sweating.

Hyperkeratosis – *h-eye-per-ke-rat-oh-sis* – excessive growth of the *stratum corneum* of the skin.

Hyperpigmentation – *h-eye-p-er-pig-men-t-ay-sh-on* – a condition of the skin, characterised by irregular patches of skin that are darker in colour than the surrounding area. It occurs when an excessive amount of *melanin* is produced in the skin. Other forms of hyperpigmentation are: *age spots* (which are caused by sun damage and are found on exposed areas of the body) and *chloasma* (large areas of darkened skin caused by hormonal change, *acne* or injury to the skin).

Hypersecretion – *h-eye-per-see-kree-sh-on* – excessive release of a substance.

Hypersensitivity – *h-eye-per-sen-sit-iv-it-ee* – over-responsiveness of the *immune system* to an external or internal stimulant (something that causes a reation), resulting in damaging reactions such as *allergies*.

Hypertension – *h-eye-per-ten-sh-on* – high *blood pressure*.

Hyperthyroidism – *h-eye-per-th-eye-roy-dis-m* – over-secretion (too much production) of *thyroxin* from the *thyroid gland* causing an increase in *metabolic rate*. Also known as an overactive thyroid gland.

Hypertrichosis – *h-eye-per-tr-eye-ko-sis* – the medical term for abnormal or excessive body hair growth in comparison to other people of the same age, sex and ethnicity. It may develop all over the body or be isolated in small areas.

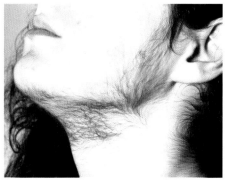

Hypertrichosis

Hypertrophy – *h-eye-per-tr-oh-fee* – an excessive enlargement or overgrowth of *tissue* that occurs without cell division, e.g. muscular hypertrophy is enlarged muscles as a result of weight training.

Hypo- – *h-eye-po* – a prefix (beginning part of a word) meaning less than normal or deficient in some way.

Hypoallergenic – *h-eye-po-al-er-jen-ik* – a common term used by the **cosmetics** industry to indicate that a product will not produce an **allergic** reaction or irritate a **sensitive skin**. Manufacturers have tried to remove as many known **allergens** and irritants from their products as possible.

Hyponychium – *h-eye-p-oh-nik-ee-um* – the skin at the end of the finger underneath the **free edge**. (See the diagram on page 190.)

Hypopigmentation – *h-eye-po-pig-men-t-ay-sh-on* – a loss of skin colour caused by a lack of **melanocytes** (the **melanin**-producing cells in the **epidermis**) or **tyrosine** (which is needed to stimulate the melanocytes to produce melanin). The most extreme form of hypopigmentation is albinisim, which is a **genetic** disorder, as there is a total lack of melanin in the skin, eyes and hair. **Vitiligo** is a condition characterised by irregular white patches of skin caused by loss of **pigment**.

Hypotension – *h-eye-po-ten-sh-on* – low **blood pressure**.

Hypothalamus – *h-eye-po-th-al-a-m-us* – part of the brain that is the control centre for the *autonomic nervous system*. It helps to regulate sleep cycles, body temperature, *blood pressure*, *metabolism*, appetite, etc. It also produces *hormones* that control the action of the *pituitary gland*.

Hypothyroidism – *h-eye-po-th-eye-roy-dis-m* – under-secretion (too little production) of *thyroxin* from the *thyroid gland* causing a decrease in *metabolic rate*. Also known as an underactive thyroid gland.

Icthyosis vulgaris – *ik-th-ee-oh-sis vul-g-ar-is* – a skin disorder characterised by persistently thick, dry, rough and flaky skin that resembles fish scales. It may be inherited or acquired in adulthood as a result of a *systemic medical condition*, *hypothyroidism*, lymphoma (a type of cancer that starts in the *lymphocytes*) or certain medications.

Identify – *eye-den-ti-f-eye* – to recognise something or someone. *Also* to recognise a need or problem and what needs to be done, e.g. the best treatment for a client.

Ileum – *il-ee-um* – the third and lowest section of the small intestine. It follows the *duodenum* and *jejunum* and is separated from the caecum (which connects the small and large intestines) by the iliocaecal *valve*.

Image – *im-a-j* – the general or public perception of a person or business, which can be good or bad. A positive image can help to promote goodwill and encourage sales.

Immune system – *im-you-n sist-em* – a complex network of organs, specialised *cells*, the *circulatory system* and the *lymphatic system* that work together to fight *infection* and defend the body from harmful substances.

Immunity – *im-you-nit-ee* – resistance to illness, *disease* or injury due to the presence of *antibodies*.

Impetigo – *im-pet-eye-go* – a common, contagious (spread by contact) skin *infection* caused by the *bacteria* Streptococcus or Staphylococcus. More common in children, it is characterised by small *blisters* that rupture (break) and form *scabs*, usually around the nose, mouth, hands and forearms, although it can affect the skin anywhere on the body.

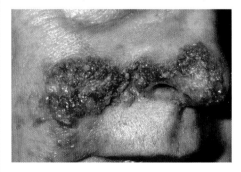

Impetigo

Improve – *im-pr-oo-v* – to make something better than it was.

Indian head massage – *in-dee-an hed mass-ar-j* – a therapeutic *treatment* based on *Ayurvedic massage* techniques, working on the upper back, shoulders, neck, scalp and face. In addition to reducing *stress*, fatigue and tension, improving mental clarity and relaxing and rejuvenating the client, it also improves the condition and health of the hair.

Induction – *in-duk-sh-on* – a special programme designed to provide new employees in a business with information about the business. This will include: the activities, products and services of the business; health and safety considerations; an outline of their job role and terms and conditions of employment; the opportunity to meet the rest of the team. The aim is to to ensure that the new employee will settle in more quickly and be confident in their new role.

Infection – *in-fek-sh-on* – invasion of a body part or tissue with a harmful *bacterium*, *fungus* or *virus*, which multiplies causing illness or damage.

Inferior – *in-f-ee-ree-or* – lower than, below, less important than. *Also* of poor quality.

Infill – *in-fil* – a procedure to fill in the gap at the base of the natural nail, when a nail extension attached to the natural nail has moved up as the nail has grown. Normally required two to three weeks after the original nail extensions have been applied.

Inflammation – *in-flam-ay-sh-on* – a reaction of the body to injury or disease, characterised by redness, swelling, heat and pain. It may be caused by the presence of *infection*, an increase in blood flow, *histamine* bathing the *tissues* or damage to the *nerve* endings.

Influence – *in-fl-oo-en-s* – the capacity or power to alter the behaviour, actions or opinions of others.

Inform – *in-for-m* – to provide information or supply knowledge to another.

Infrared – *in-f-r-a red* – *radiation* in the invisible part of the *electromagnetic spectrum* with *wavelengths* greater than 760 nanometres (760 thousand-millionths of a metre).

Ingestion – *in-jest-yon* – taking food into the body via the *digestive system*.

Ingrown hair – *in-gr-oh-n h-air* – a hair that curls and penetrates the skin with its tip. It may become inflamed and can be caused by very dry skin, stiff beard hair, build-up of dead skin cells in the *hair follicle* and on the surface of the skin, or coarse, curly hair growing in a curved follicle. Hair removal methods such as waxing, plucking, shaving or electrolysis often irritate the follicle.

Ingrown nail – *in-gr-oh-n n-ay-l* – see *onychocryptosis*.

Inhale – *in-hay-l* – to breathe air into the body. This occurs when the *diaphragm* contracts, moving downward and expanding the chest cavity, allowing air to flow into the lungs.

Inner root sheath – *in-er r-oo-t sh-ee-th* – the innermost part of the *hair follicle*, with three layers: Henle's layer, which is one cell thick; Huxley's layer, which is two or more cells thick; and the *cuticle*.

Innervation – *in-er-vay-sh-on* – distribution or supply of *nerves* to a part of the body.

Insertion – *in-s-er-sh-on* – the end of a *muscle* attached to a freely moving bone, the moveable point on which the force of the muscle is applied.

Insulin – *in-s-you-lin* – a *hormone* produced by the *pancreas* in the *Islets of Langerhans*. It regulates *carbohydrate metabolism* and is required by the *cells* of the body to remove and use *glucose* from the blood.

Insurance – *in-sh-or-an-s* – the payment of a fixed sum of money on a regular basis to a company which will then pay an agreed sum in the event of injury, illness, loss or damage. There are many types of insurance a business must consider, some of which are *professional indemnity*, *public* *liability*, *product liability*, health, fire and car insurance.

Integumentary system – *in-teg-you-men-t-a-ree sis-tem* – the system of the body consisting of the skin, hair and nails.

Intense pulsed light (IPL) – *in-ten-s pul-s-d l-eye-t* – an electrical therapy using a special lamp which directs pulses (bursts) of light onto the skin to penetrate through the upper layers. It stimulates new *collagen* and *elastin* to improve skin health, it reduces the appearance of blemishes and scar tissue, evens out colouring and is also used for hair removal.

Intensity – *in-ten-sit-ee* – strength or concentration.

Intercellular fluid – *in-t-er-sel-you-l-er fl-oo-id* – see *tissue fluid*.

Intercellular matrix – *in-t-er-sel-you-l-er may-tr-ix* – a combination of substances that acts as 'mortar' holding the layers of skin cells together and creating a natural barrier to keep *bacteria* out and moisture in.

Intercostal muscles – *in-t-er-kos-t-l mus-sel-s* – small *muscles* between the *ribs*. The internal intercostals aid in breathing out by pulling down the ribs and reducing the size of the thoracic (chest) cavity. The external intercostals help when breathing in as they raise the ribs and increase the dimensions of the thoracic cavity.

Interstitial fluid – *in-ter-st-i-sh-l fl-oo-id* – see *tissue fluid*.

Introduce – *in-tr-o-d-yoo-s* – to present one person to another. *Also* to bring to someone's attention a new experience that they have not tried before, or to demonstrate and *promote* the latest technology to clientele.

Involuntary muscle – *in-vol-un-ta-r-ee mus-sel* – a *muscle* that contracts without conscious control, found in the walls of internal organs such as the stomach, intestine and bladder and in *blood vessels*.

Ion – *eye-on* – an electrically charged *atom* formed by the loss or gain of one or more *electrons*.

Ionisation – *eye-on-eye-zay-sh-on* – the use of active *ions* in galvanic facial and body treatments (see *galvanic unit*).

Iontophoresis – *eye-on-tof-or-ee-sis* – introduction of ionised products (see *ionisation*) into the skin using a *galvanic current*. It can be used to improve all skin conditions.

Irradiation – *i-ray-dee-ay-sh-on* – the emission (sending out) of rays of light, heat or other form of energy.

Irritation – *i-rit-ay-sh-on* – a condition of soreness or *inflammation* in the body or on the skin.

Islets of Langerhans – *eye-let-s of lan-ger-hans* – the *hormone*-producing *cells* of the *pancreas* that secrete (release) *insulin*, *glucagon* and somatostatin (which inhibits the release of certain other hormones), directly into the blood flow.

Jacuzzi – *jak-oo-z-ee* – the name given to a whirlpool bath or spa, after the man who invented it, Roy Jacuzzi, in 1968.

Jejunum – *je-joo-num* – the middle part of the small intestine between the **duodenum** and the **ileum**.

Jewellery – *j-oo-el-er-ee* – any personal items of adornment, including earrings, necklaces, body piercing and bracelets. They must be removed prior to **treatment**, particularly when using electrical equipment.

Job description – *job des-krip-shon* – a clear outline of a job role, produced when a new member of staff is required. It is used to set out the roles and responsibilities of the successful candidate, provide the information for drawing up a **person specification** and supply details for the job advertisement. It allows the candidate to consider whether they have the necessary skills and requirements to do the job.

Job role – *job r-oh-l* – the actions, activities and responsibilities involved in carrying out a position of employment.

Job title – *job t-eye-t-l* – the name that describes the position of an employee in a business and what they do.

Joint – *joy-n-t* – the point at which two bones are connected.

Jojoba oil – *ho-ho-ba oy-l* – a liquid used as a **carrier oil** in aromatherapy. It closely resembles the skin's own **sebum**, making it ideal for all **skin types**. It has **anti-inflammatory** and **antioxidant** effects and mixes well with other carrier oils.

Joule – *j-oo-l* – a unit of electrical energy equal to the work done when a current of one **ampere** is passed through a resistance of one **ohm** for one second.

Junior therapist – *j-oo-nee-or th-e-rap-is-t* – the least experienced member of a team of therapists, who provides support and assistance to more senior therapists.

Kaolin – *k-ay-oh-lin* – very fine white clay included as a light-diffusing (spreading light) ingredient in **cosmetics** and as an ingredient in **face masks**. It is used for its cleansing effect and the ability to draw impurities from the skin.

Keloid – *k-ee-l-oy-d* – a raised formation of **scar** tissue caused by excessive **tissue** repair in response to trauma or surgery. The **fibroblasts** continue to multiply and form large mounds of scar tissue. **Black skins** are more susceptible to keloid formation.

Keratin – *ke-rat-in* – a **protein** produced by **keratinocytes** and found in hair, the outer layer of skin and nails.

Keratinisation – *ke-rat-in-eye-say-shon* – the process by which **keratin** is deposited in cells and the cells become horny, as in nails and hair, providing a waterproof barrier.

Keratinocytes – *k-e-rat-in-oh-s-eye-t-s* – cells that make up the **epidermis**, which produce a **protein** called **keratin**. (See the diagram on page 189.)

Keratolytic – *ke-rat-o-lit-ik* – a substance that causes the loosening or shedding of the **stratum corneum** of the skin.

Kinesis – *kin-ee-sis* – movement or activity in response to a stimulus (something that provokes a reaction).

Kneading – *need-in-g* – a **massage** manipulation that involves compressing and releasing muscle tissues against each other or against underlying bone, performed with either or both hands. It can be alternate (one hand at a time) or reinforced (one hand on top of the other) and can be adapted for different parts of the body, to take in to account differences in the shape and size of muscles. The whole of the palmar (front) surface of the hands is used, pressing the muscles gently against underlying structures in a circular movement. It may be modified by using the pads of the thumbs and the first and second fingers.

Kneipp therapy – *n-ee-p th-er-rap-ee* – a water **therapy** originating in Germany and developed by Sebastian Kneipp, a priest and naturopath (someone who practises natural remedies, e.g. water and heat therapies and massage). The method incorporates immersion (being placed into water either partially or totally) into very cold and hot water alternately to stimulate the circulation and strengthen the *immune system*.

Knuckling – *nuk-lin-g* – a *kneading* massage manipulation classified as *frictions*. It is performed with the hand curled into a loose fist, moving in small circular strokes and used on areas such as the shoulders and chest.

Koilonychia – *k-oy-lon-ik-ee-a* – abnormally shaped nails that are thin and concave with raised *lateral* and *distal* edges. It may be caused by iron deficiency, i.e. *anaemia*, Raynaud's disease (a condition in which blood supply to the fingers and toes is reduced) or direct trauma (injury) to the nail. Also known as spoon-shaped nails.

Kyphosis – *k-eye-foh-sis* – an abnormal outward curvature of the spine causing a hunchback.

Laconium – *lak-oh-nee-um* – a dry, gentle **sauna** treatment originating in the **spas** of ancient Rome. It is used before further **heat treatment** to gently open the **pores** in a temperature of around 65°C and a low humidity of around 15–20 per cent.

Lactic acid – *lak-tik as-id* – a substance formed from **glucose** and used by **muscles** for energy.

Lamella dystrophy – *lam-el-a dis-tr-of-ee* – flaking, peeling and breaking of the **nail plate**. It has many causes, including exposure to harsh chemicals, poor **diet**, overuse of false nails, general ill-health, immersing hands in water for long periods, incorrect filing, excessive **buffing**, neglect and using the nails as tools.

Lanolin – *lan-o-lin* – comes from the **sebaceous glands** of sheep and closely resembles the oil from human sebaceous glands. It is an effective moisturising agent but has a reputation as an **allergen** for some skins.

Lanugo hair – *lan-you-go h-air* – a coat of delicate, downy hairs covering the human foetus (unborn baby).

Laser – *l-ay-s-er* – stands for **l**ight **a**mplification **s**timulated **e**mission **r**adiation. This is an increasingly popular specialised **treatment**, used to improve skin texture and to reduce fine lines and **wrinkles** and **superfluous** hair on the body and face. Lasers are used by dermatologists (doctors specialising in skin

Langerhans' cells – *lan-ger-han-s sels* – found in the **stratum spinosum** of the **epidermis**, these cells are responsible for starting an immune response in the body to fight **infection** and destroy certain foreign (from outside the body) substances.

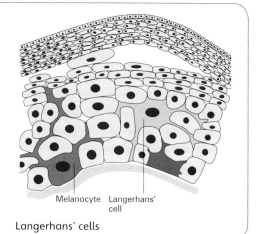

Melanocyte Langerhans' cell

Langerhans' cells

complaints) for some skin conditions such as *port wine stains*, dilated (enlarged) *blood vessels*, and removal of birthmarks, tattoos, *warts* and *skin tags*.

Lateral – *lat-er-al* – positioned away from the *midline* of the body, towards the side.

Latissimus dorsi – *lat-is-im-us d-or-s-eye* – a large, triangular, flat *muscle* on each side of the back, covering the lumbar (lower back) area and the lower half of the thoracic (chest) area. It extends, adducts (moves inwards) and rotates the arm inwards and draws the shoulder down and backwards.

Laws – *l-or-s* – principles and regulations established in a community (e.g. a country) by an authority (e.g. a government) and which apply to all the people in the community. Laws must be obeyed and are enforced by the courts of law.

Legal – *l-ee-g-al* – permitted by law.

Legionnaires' disease – *lee-jon-er-s dis-ee-s* – an illness

caused by inhaling droplets of water suspended in air that are infected with a *bacterium* called *Legionella pneumophilia*. Outbreaks occur in places with purpose-built water systems where temperatures are warm enough to encourage growth of the bacteria, such as whirlpool spas, cooling towers and air conditioning and industrial cooling systems.

Legislation – *lej-is-lay-shon* – a *law* or body of laws that affects the way in which a business is run and how services are delivered to clients. Legislation is designed to protect the business owner as well as the client.

Lentigo – *len-ti-go* (plural **lentigines** – *len-ti-jee-ns*) – a type of *freckle*. Lentigo simplex may be present at birth but usually develops in early childhood. Solar lentigo is another term for *age spots*.

Lesion – *lee-shon* – a wound or injury or an abnormal change in *tissue* formation, usually caused by trauma (injury), *infection*, damage or *disease*.

Leucocyte – *loo-ko-site* – see *white blood cell*.

Leucoderma – *loo-ko-der-ma* – see *vitiligo*.

Leuconychia – *loo-kon-ik-ee-a* – white spots appearing on the *nail plate* which will eventually grow out, caused by air bubbles or a blow to the nail.

Levator labii – *le-v-ay-t-or lab-ee-eye* – a facial *muscle* situated between the side of the nose and the *zygomatic bone* which raises the upper lip. Some people call it the 'Elvis muscle' because of the expressive snarl made famous by Elvis Presley. (See the diagram on page 192.)

Levator palpabrae – *le-v-ay-t-or pal-p-br-ay* – the *muscle* of the eyelid, the action of which is to raise the eyelid. (See the diagram on page 192.)

Licence – *l-eye-sen-s* – a legal document giving permission or authorisation for a specific activity, such as to manufacture, use or sell a certain product.

Lifestyle – *l-eye-f-st-eye-l* – a way of life. The habits, attitudes, standards, economic level and tastes that reflect the style of living of a person or group. Information about a client's lifestyle will help the therapist develop an appropriate *treatment plan*. Lifestyle advice is also an important aspect of the complete treatment, as suggestions concerning changes in lifestyle may improve the results achieved.

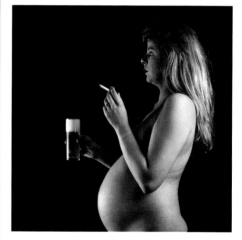

Changes in lifestyle can increase the effectiveness of a treatment and health of the client

Ligament – *lig-a-men-t* – *connective tissue* attaching bone to bone.

Limbic system – *lim-bik sis-t-em* – part of the human brain that deals with emotion, memory and motivation.

Limited company – *lim-it-ed com-pan-ee* – a legal business status, in which the company's finances are separate from the personal finances of the owners. The shareholders' personal assets are protected if the business fails. A private limited company may have one or more members but cannot offer shares to the public. A public limited company (PLC) must have at least two shareholders and may offer shares to the public. A limited company must be registered at Companies House and must have at least one director (two if it is a PLC) and a company secretary, who may also be shareholders. From October 2008, it will no longer be necessary for PLCs to have a company secretary.

Link selling – *lin-k sel-lin-g* – to make a sale by providing goods that relate to or complement others, e.g. if a client is buying a *cleanser* they may also wish to buy the *toning lotion* or *moisturiser* that complement it. Other examples are a nail enamel in a particular colour to match a lipstick or a scented bubble bath or body lotion to match a perfume.

Lip balm – *lip b-ar-m* – a softening and moisturising product for the lips to prevent them chapping and to protect them from the environment. The lips have no sweat *glands* or *sebaceous glands* and therefore dry out very easily.

Lip gloss – *lip g-loss* – a cosmetic used to provide shine and colour to the lips. It comes in two forms: a viscous (thick) liquid or a soft solid. Other ingredients such as *collagen* and plumping agents are added to *enhance* the texture and appearance of the lips. It is applied with a brush or wand or squeezed from a tube directly onto the lips.

Lipliner – *lip l-eye-n-er* – a cosmetic lip pencil used to provide definition to the lips or change the shape of the mouth before applying *lipstick*. A hard pencil will prevent the lipstick 'bleeding' into the fine lines around the mouth.

Liposomes – *lip-o-so-m-s* – microscopic (cannot be seen with the naked eye) fluid-filled *(continued)*

101

sacs within cosmetics, used to deliver substances into the skin. They hold the ingredients and then release them after being absorbed into the skin.

Lipstick – *lip st-ik* – a cosmetic product used to add colour and moisture to the lips. It contains a mixture of oils, waxes, *pigments* and *emollients* and is best applied with a lip brush.

Liquefying cleanser – *lik-w-f-eye-in-g klen-s-er* – a *cleansing cream* with a high oil content that melts when applied to the skin. It removes all traces of *makeup* and leaves the skin moist and supple without upsetting the *acid mantle*.

Lordosis – *l-or-d-oh-sis* – an abnormal forward curvature of the spine in the lumbar (lower back) region. Also known as swayback or saddle back.

Lumbar – *lum-bar* – the area of the back between the lowest *ribs* and the hips.

Lumen – *loo-men* – the space inside a tube within the body, e.g. inside a *blood vessel*.

Lunula – *loo-n-you-la* – see *half moon*.

Luteinising hormone (LH) – *l-oo-ten-eye-s-in-g h-or-m-oh-n* – a *hormone* secreted (released) by the **anterior** lobe (section) of the *pituitary gland*. In the female it stimulates the ovary to release the ovum (egg) and prepares the *uterus* to receive the fertilised egg. In the male it stimulates the *testes* to produce *testosterone*.

Lye – *l-eye* – another name for sodium hydroxide, which is formed when the salts of the body separate and reform when in contact with *direct current*.

Lymph – *lim-f* – the fluid in the *lymphatic system*, which comes from blood *plasma*. It circulates around the lymphatic system removing *bacteria* and certain *proteins* from the *tissues*. It also transports fat from the small intestine to the blood and supplies mature *lymphocytes* to the blood. Lymph flows from the tissues to the *lymph nodes*, then to the right *lymphatic duct* and the *thoracic duct*, and from there lymph drains into the right and left subclavian veins (see *lymph drainage*).

Lymph capillaries – *lim-f kap-il-a-r-ee-s* – tiny channels with thin walls through which **nutrients**, dissolved gases and waste products can easily pass. They are the main area of **exchange** between the **lymph** that bathes the body **tissues** and the blood.

Lymph drainage – *lim-f dr-ay-n-aj* – the movement of **lymph** from the body's **tissues**, through the **lymph vessels**, to the **lymph nodes**, cleansing the tissues. This is done by returning the lymph to the **circulatory system** from the right **lymphatic duct** and the **thoracic duct** via the subclavian veins (part of the network of major **veins** of the upper body – the left subclavian vein receives lymph from the thoracic duct). Lymph drainage may be increased using mechanical or manual **massage**. Mechanical massage techniques include **vacuum suction**, G5 (a vibratory massage treatment) or Endermologie® (a treatment for **cellulite**). Manual lymph drainage massage uses gentle, wave-like movements to drain away excess fluid and trapped **toxins**.

Lymph nodes – *lim-f n-oh-d-s* – small structures made of **lymphatic tissue**, located at intervals along the **lymphatic system**, particularly at the neck, under the arm and in the groin. They filter **bacteria** and foreign (from outside the body) particles from **lymph** fluid. When the body is fighting infection lymph nodes may become swollen with activated **lymphocytes**. (See the diagram on page 199.)

Lymph vessels – *lim-f ve-sel-s* – channels or ducts in the **lymphatic system** that contain and carry lymph from the **tissues** to the **circulatory system**. The walls are thin and they contain **valves** that prevent **lymph** from flowing backwards. (See the diagram on page 199.) Also known as lymphatics.

Lymphatic duct – *lim-fat-ik d-uk-t* – part of the **lymphatic system** – the right lymphatic duct and the **thoracic duct** are channels that drain **lymph** fluid into the **circulatory system**. (See the diagram on page 199.)

Lymphatic organs – *lim-fat-ik or-g-an-s* – specialised groups of **lymphatic tissue** which include: the **thymus gland**; the spleen (the largest of the lymphatic *(continued)* organs, situated in the upper left part of the *abdomen*, which filters blood, acts as a blood reservoir (store) and destroys old blood cells); and the tonsils (small masses of lymphatic tissue situated on either side at the back of the throat). (See the diagram on page 199.)

Lymphatic system – *lim-f-at-ik sis-t-em* – the system through which *lymph* circulates around the body to protect it from *disease*, clean it of waste and maintain fluid balance. It consists of *lymph*, *lymph vessels*, *lymph nodes*, *lymphatic ducts*, the *thymus gland*, spleen, tonsils and bone

marrow. (See the diagram on page 199.)

Lymphatic tissue – *lim-fat-ik ti-sh-you* – a special type of *connective tissue* containing large numbers of *lymphocytes*. It forms the *thymus gland*, the spleen and the tonsils.

Lymphocytes – *lim-f-oh-s-eye-t-s* – *white blood cells* produced in the bone marrow. Known as B cells (because they remain in the bone marrow to mature) and T cells (see *thymus gland*), they are transported around the body in the *circulatory* and *lymphatic systems* carrying out activities in the *immune system*.

Macadamia oil – *mak-a-dee-me-a oy-l* – a **carrier oil** used in **aromatherapy** that contains high amounts of a fatty acid also found in **sebum**. This oil therefore has similarities with the natural oil in human skin and is good for **dry skin**.

Maceration – *mas-er-ay-sh-on* – a method of extracting **essential oils** from flowers using hot oil. The flowers are soaked in the oil and their **cell membranes** rupture (break), releasing the **essential oil**. The fragrant oil is then decanted (poured into another container) ready for use.

Macrophages – *mak-r-oh-f-ay-j* – part of the **immune system**. A type of **white blood cell** capable of ingesting (absorbing) micro-organisms (tiny organisms that can't be seen with the naked eye), dead cells and foreign particles in a process known as phagocytosis.

Macule – *mak-you-l* – a pigmented (coloured) area of the skin that is not raised above the surface.

Magnesium carbonate – *mag-nee-zee-um k-ar-bon-ay-t* – a light, white powder with absorbent properties, used in **cosmetics** and as an ingredient in **face masks**.

Magnifying light – *mag-ni-f-eye-in-g l-eye-t* – a special glass lens with a light attached. When viewed through the lens, the size of an object appears increased and clarity is improved. The lens provides a more detailed view and is useful when **analysing** the skin before treatment or when providing a service such as **epilation** that requires accuracy and careful probing.

Maintain – *m-ay-n-t-ay-n* – to keep in good condition for use.

Makeup – *m-ay-k-up* – **cosmetics** used to **enhance**, change or camouflage (hide or disguise) the appearance, used on the face or body. In the salon, makeup is applied for different occasions: day, evening, bridal, party, photographic, camouflaging tattoos, catwalk or theatrical. The makeup chosen should complement the client's colouring, be suitable for the occasion, coordinate with clothes and accessories and suit the client's **skin type**.

Male skin – *m-ay-l sk-in* – this has a thicker *epidermis* than female skin, approximately 20% thicker, as it contains more *elastin* and *collagen*. It produces more *sweat* and *sebum* and is prone to *comedones*, razor bumps and *ingrown hairs* in the beard area. Quite often it will be sensitive (see *sensitive skin*), particularly after shaving, which can also have a dehydrating effect (see *dehydrated skin*).

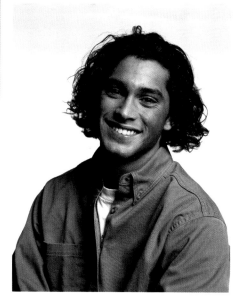

Male skin has a thicker epidermis than female skin

Malignant – *mal-ig-nan-t* – dangerous or harmful. A malignant disorder is one which may become life threatening unless treated. Most often used to describe cancer.

Malignant melanoma – *mal-ig-nan-t mel-a-no-ma* – a cancer of the *melanocytes* in the *epidermis*. Most common in *white skin*, the main risk factors in developing melanoma are sun exposure (particularly in childhood), sunburn that causes *blisters* (especially when young), fair skin that burns easily, previous melanoma, family history, large numbers of *moles* (especially in excess of 100) and abnormal moles.

Manager – *man-a j-er* – a person who has control of resources and expenditure and directs the employees and activities of a business or a department within a business.

Mandible – *man-dib-l* – the fusion of two bones (two bones joined together) that forms the lower jaw. The mandible holds the lower teeth. (See the diagram on page 196.)

Manicure – *man-ik-y-or* – a cosmetic (designed to improve the appearance) *treatment* of the hands and fingernails which includes filing, *cuticle* care, *massage* and enamelling.

Manufacturer – *man-you-fak-t-y-or* – a person, group or company that makes goods.

Market niche – *mar-k-et n-ee-sh* – a segment of the potential clients of a business. Specific services and products can be aimed at a market niche – e.g. offering ecofriendly products for people who want to protect the environment.

Market segmentation – *mar-k-et seg-men-tay-sh-on* – breaking the potential clients of a business into groups with similar characteristics, who can be targeted for different products or services.

Marketing – *mar-ket-in-g* – the process involved in identifying consumer requirements and making clients aware of the products and services available.

Marma pressure points – *m-ar-ma pre-sh-or p-oy-n-t-s* – part of the Ayurvedic system of medicine (see *Ayurveda*), these are 107 points in the body occurring where **blood vessels**, **ligaments** and **nerve** centres join. The points correspond to internal organs and systems and can be massaged to release blocked energy, restore normal function and energise or relax. Marma pressure point *massage* was originally used in ancient India for self-defence, healing and to increase flexibility in martial arts.

Mascara – *mas-k-ar-a* – a cosmetic used to darken and thicken the eyelashes, providing definition to the eyes. It comes in several forms – cream, liquid and block – as well as a variety of colours. It is applied to the lashes with a brush or wand and contains *wax* thickeners, film formers (ingredients that form a covering over the hair), *emollients* and preservatives. It can also contain rayon or nylon fibres to add length.

Massage – *mas-ar-j* – manual manipulation (movement) of the skin and **muscles** for a therapeutic purpose using different techniques. There are many different types of massage including: **Swedish**, **aromatherapy**, **lymph drainage**, Tui Na (Chinese medical massage), Lomi Lomi (from Hawaii), **hot stone**, neuromuscular, rolfing (deep tissue massage), shiatsu (a type of acupressure), **Thai** and Balinese. Most types of massage, and in particular Swedish massage, include **effleurage**, **petrissage**, **percussion** and **vibrations** as part of the routine. Massage should be smooth and rhythmical with an even depth and pressure, which may be adapted for the size and condition of the client.

Massage cream – *mas-ar-j kr-ee-m* – an **emollient** used to moisturise the skin. It is an ideal massage medium for hairy skin. Cream is absorbed into the skin more quickly than oil.

Massage medium – *mass-ar-j m-ee-dee-um* – a lubricant (a substance used to allow ease of movement) such as oil, cream, powder or lotion used during body and facial **massage**. The massage medium should be used sparingly and applied from the therapist's hands, not directly from the container onto the client's skin. The choice of medium depends on client preference, type of massage and **skin type**.

Masseter – *ma-see-t-er* – a short, powerful **muscle** in the lower cheek that closes the jaw and helps with chewing. (See the diagram on page 192.)

Mast cells – *ma-s-t sel-s* – part of the **immune system**. These **cells** originate in bone marrow (soft tissue inside the bones) and settle in **connective tissue** where they release substances in response to **inflammation** of body tissues from injury or **allergic** reaction. When activated, they release **histamine** and heparin among other things. Histamine causes swelling and itching of the affected tissue; heparin prevents harmful clots forming.

Matrix – *m-ay-tr-ix* – the root of the nail, which produces cells that form the **nail plate**. Also the lower part of the **hair bulb** where cells multiply and form the hair.

Matte polish – *mat po-li-sh* – enamel or varnish applied to the nails to provide a non-shiny finish. Popular in a male manicure and for females who do not want colour.

Mature skin – *mat-y-or s-k-in* – a *skin type* that is dry and tight with a dull appearance. It is no longer supple and there is a loss of *muscle tone*. *Wrinkles* are evident and there may be uneven pigmentation (colouring). It is caused by a lack of moisture, a decrease in *sebum* flow and reduced *collagen* and *elastin* production, all of which are normal effects of ageing.

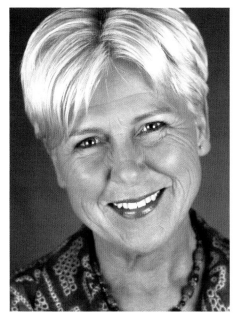

Mature skin type

Maxilla – *max-ill-a* – the fusion of two bones (joining together) that forms the upper jaw. The maxilla holds the upper teeth. (See the diagram on page 196.)

Medi spa – *med-ee sp-ar* – an establishment that provides both medical treatments and *spa therapies*.

Medial – *mee-dee-al* – situated in the middle or towards the *midline* of the body.

Medical referral – *med-ik-al r-fer-al* – recommending a person to seek advice from a general practitioner (GP).

Medical spa – *med-ik-l sp-ar* – a *day spa* or *destination spa* that provides traditional and complementary medical services, administered or supervised by medical professionals. Treatments may include diagnostic, preventative and cosmetic techniques.

Medicated cleanser – *med-ik-ay-ted klen-s-er* – a *cleanser* containing ingredients to counteract (work against) bacterial infection of the skin.

Mediterranean skin – *med-it-er-ay-nee-an s-k-in* – this *skin type* has a combination of both red and yellow *pigment* that provides the typical olive colour. It is usually oily but not prone to spots or *acne*. It ages better than *white skin* and is protected from damage from *ultraviolet radiation* by its ability to tan quickly without burning. A problem for this skin type is sometimes an excess of facial hair, which can be coarser and darker than that of other skin types.

Medulla – *med-u-la* – the inner core of certain organs or body structures, e.g. the hair and the *adrenal gland*. (See the diagram on page 191.)

Melanin – *me-la-n-in* – a *pigment* found in skin and hair. Produced by special skin cells (*melanocytes*) that are sensitive to sunlight, melanin protects the body by absorbing *ultraviolet radiation* from the sun. The amount of melanin present determines the colour of a person's complexion: people with a large amount have darker skin, whereas people with very little have fair skin. Melanin also determines the colour of the iris in the eyes.

Melanocyte – *mel-an-oh-s eye-t* – a *pigment* cell in the *stratum germinativum* of the *epidermis* that produces *melanin* to protect the skin from *ultraviolet radiation*.

Melanocyte stimulating hormone – *mel-an-oh-s-eye-t st-im-you-lay-tin-g hor-m-oh-n* – a chemical made by the *anterior* lobe (section) of the *pituitary gland*. It stimulates the production and release of *melanin* by the *melanocytes* in the skin and hair. The level of this *hormone* increases during pregnancy and, together with an increase in *oestrogen*, this may cause increased pigmentation (colouring) in the skin.

Melanosomes – *mel-an-oh-soh-m-s* – coloured *melanin* granules in the skin that provide the different shades of colour. In *black skin*, these granules are larger and heavily pigmented (coloured) and in white skin they are smaller and contain less melanin.

Melatonin – *mel-at-oh-nin* – a *hormone* secreted (released) by the *pineal gland*. Its production is stimulated (increased) by darkness and inhibited (slowed down) by light. It reaches its peak in the middle of the night and then gradually starts to fall. Its function is to regulate the sleep patterns in the body.

Membrane – *mem-b-ray-n* – a thin, flexible sheet of *tissue* that lines organs or connects body parts.

Menopause – *men-oh-p-or-s* – the end of the *menstrual cycle*, the last menstrual period. This occurs naturally when the *ovaries* stop producing the *hormones oestrogen* and *progesterone*. The average age of the menopause is 51. It also occurs after chemotherapy or radiotherapy or when the ovaries are removed through surgery.

Menstrual cycle – *men-st-roo-al s-eye-k-l* – a recurring sequence of physiological (involving normal functioning of the body systems) changes in the female, associated with fertility (ability to conceive and have children). It includes the release of ova (eggs) from the *ovaries* and *menstruation*.

Menstruation – *men-st-r-oo-ay-sh-on* – part of the *menstrual cycle* in which the *endometrium* is shed once a month, resulting in blood flow from the vagina.

Mentalis – *men-tar-lis* – a small facial *muscle* situated at the tip of the chin. It raises and pushes up the lower lip, causing wrinkling of the lip, as in expressing displeasure. (See the diagram on page 192.)

Mesomorph – *mee-so-mor-f* – a strong, muscular body type, angular with broad shoulders and narrow hips, usually well muscled and with little body fat.

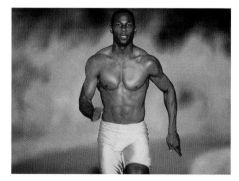

The mesomorph body type

Message – *mes-a-j* – a short communication sent by words, signals or other means from one person to another.

Metabolic rate – *met-ab-ol-ik r-ay-t* – the speed of *metabolism*, how quickly the body burns fuel and transforms it into energy.

Metabolic waste – *met-ab-ol-ik w-ay-st* – substances produced by *metabolism* that are not wanted by the body and need to be eliminated (got rid of), e.g. *carbon dioxide*, nitrogen compounds, excess water, phosphates and sulphates.

Metabolism – *met-ab-oh-lis-m* – the chemical processes that take place in the *cells* of the body, by which energy is produced and substances are synthesised (combined) for growth and repair.

Metatarsals – *met-at-ar-sal-s* – the five long bones in the foot connected to the ankle bones. (See the diagram on page 197.)

Microamp – *my-kr-oh-amp* – a unit of electricity, one millionth of an *ampere*.

Microcurrent – *my-kr-oh-ku-r-en-t* – low-frequency, modified *direct current*, which is much smaller than any other current used in therapeutic *treatment*. This type of current is thought to resemble closely the natural bio-electrical (describing the electric current generated by living tissue) impulses of the body. It is used in the popular 'non-surgical facelift' to tighten and firm facial and body contours and aid *lymph drainage*.

Microcurrent unit – *my-kr-oh-ku-r-en-t yoo-nit* – the machine used to provide a tightening, lifting, firming *treatment* using a *microcurrent*. It also helps to improve skin condition, in particular reducing fine lines, *scar* and stretch marks.

Microdermabrasion – *my-kr-oh-der-ma-br-ay-sh-on* – a cosmetic procedure developed in Italy in 1985, in which the *stratum corneum* is partially removed using mechanical *abrasion* from jets of zinc oxide or aluminium oxide crystals. It is used to remove sun-damaged skin, and to reduce fine lines and lessen *scars*, stretch marks and *hyperpigmentation*. It is a popular treatment for clients who do not want the higher-risk treatments such as standard dermabrasion, *chemical peeling* or *laser* resurfacing.

Midline – *mid-l-eye-n* – an imaginary line down the centre of the body used to describe positions in the body and muscle actions.

Milium – *mil-ee-um (plural* **milia** – *mil-ee-a)* – a tiny white or yellowish bump just underneath the surface of the skin caused by skin cells covering the mouth of the *follicle* and trapping *sebum* from the *sebaceous gland*. Also known as a *whitehead*.

Milliampere – *mil-ee-am-p-er* – a unit of electricity, one thousandth of an *ampere*.

Mineral makeup – *min-er-al may-k-up* – made from minerals and *pigments* that have been micropulverised (ground down to the smallest possible size), this type of *makeup* has an ultra-fine powder formulation, is water-resistant and has staying power, with no added *preservatives*, talc, oil or *fragrances*. It provides excellent skin coverage and is suitable for all *skin types* and ages.

Mineral oil – *min-er-al oy-l* – a clear, odourless oil derived from petroleum and widely used in *cosmetics* as it rarely causes *allergic* reactions and does not become solid and block *pores*.

Mitosis – *my-toe-sis* – the process of cell division in which the *nucleus* divides and two identical cells are produced.

Modesty – *mod-es-t-ee* – shyness or decency in speech, dress or behaviour.

Modification to treatment – *mod-if-ik-ay-sh-on to tr-ee-t-men-t* – an alteration, adaptation or change in the *treatment* to suit the client's needs. This may be because the client has a bad back, is pregnant, elderly or disabled, and may therefore need additional support when lying or for treatment to be performed in a sitting position. Certain aspects of the treatment may be changed in some way, e.g. reducing the intensity of an *electric current*, removing certain movements from a procedure or avoiding certain products in order to avoid an *allergic* reaction.

Moisturiser – *m-oy-st-your-eyes-er* – a cosmetic product designed to hydrate and lubricate (oil) the outer layers of the skin, to keep it soft and supple and prevent further moisture loss. There are many types of moisturiser available and they may include ingredients such as *humectants* that attract water from the atmosphere, *occlusives* that provide an oily barrier on the skin to prevent moisture loss and other *emollients* such as *lanolin* and *glycerine*. Moisturisers come in different formulations: creams, lotions, milks, special night creams, eye and neck creams. They are also effective in providing a smooth base over which *makeup* is applied and they may be translucent (semi-transparent) or coloured to suit different skin tones or used as a light covering for people who do not like to wear *foundation*.

Mole – *m-oh-l* – a *benign* growth on the skin, which may be raised or flat, pigmented (coloured) or skin coloured.

Molecule – *mol-ek-you-l* – a chemical combination of two or more *atoms*.

Monitor – *mon-it-or* – to observe, oversee, supervise or regulate, e.g. a business, procedure or people. *Also* the small screen on a computer or other piece of equipment, which provides information for the operator.

Monomer – *mon-o-mer* – a small *molecule* that may become chemically bonded to other monomers to form a *polymer*.

Motor nerve – *m-oh-tor n-er-v* – an *efferent* nerve carrying impulses (messages) from the *central nervous system* to *muscles* or organs. It stimulates movement in muscles and stimulates *glands* to secrete (release) *hormones*.

Motor point – *m-oh-tor p-oy-n-t* – the part of a *muscle* where the *nerve* enters and when stimulated by a *faradic current* produces movement of the muscle.

Multiple sclerosis – *m-ul-tip-l sk-ler-oh-sis* – an *autoimmune disease* that affects the *central nervous system*. It is believed to be caused by damage to the protective covering of the *neurons*.

Muscle – *m-us-sel* – tissue in the body that is capable of contracting (shortening and tightening), the function of which is to produce force and cause movement. Muscle **contraction** is both voluntary (under the person's conscious control), to move the body, and involuntary (happens automatically), which is necessary for survival, e.g. contraction of the **heart** to pump blood and **peristalsis** (the movement of food during **digestion**).

Muscle fatigue – *mus-sel fat-ee-g* – a decrease in the ability of a **muscle** to create force when it becomes tired after physical exertion.

Muscle tone – *mus-sel toe-n* – the ability of muscles to respond to a stretch. *Also* the state of permanent partial **contraction** of the muscles which helps the body maintain its **posture**.

Muscular dystrophy – *mus-q-lar dis-tro-f-ee* – a disorder that causes progressive **muscle** weakness and loss of muscle **tissue**.

Muscular endurance – *mus-q-lar end-your-an-s* – the ability of

a **muscle** to repeatedly exert force or to maintain a fixed **contraction** for a period of time.

Muscular strength – *mus-q-lar st-ren-g-th* – the ability of the body's **muscles** to generate extreme amounts of force in a short period using **anaerobic** (without oxygen) energy.

Muscular system – *mus-q-lar sis-tem* – the **muscles** of the body, composed of specialised muscle **tissue** that contracts (shortens and tightens) to produce movement in the body. It contains both voluntary **skeletal muscles** attached to bones (which produce conscious movement) and involuntary **smooth muscles** (which make up the internal vessels and organs such as **arteries**, **veins**, digestive tract (see **peristalsis**) and urinary bladder). **Cardiac muscle** is only found in the **heart** and its function is to pump blood through the **circulatory system**. It is an **involuntary muscle** (contracting without direct control by the **nervous system**). (See the diagram on page 198.)

Myelin sheath – *m-eye-e-lin sh-ee-th* – an insulating (doesn't conduct electricity) layer formed around **nerves** to allow the rapid transmission (sending) of nerve impulses (signals) along the **neurons**.

Naevus – *n-ee-v-us* (plural **naevi** – *nee-v-eye*) – a congenital (present at birth) pigmented (coloured) area of skin. It results from an excess of pigmentation, the exaggerated development of blood vessels or an overgrowth of *epidermal tissue* or *connective tissue*. Birthmarks and *moles* are both types of naevi.

Nail – *n-ay-l* – a protective covering for the ends of the fingers and toes. It is composed of a *nail bed*, nail *matrix* and *nail plate*. Finger nails grow at the rate of 0.1 millimetre per day, whereas toe nails grow more slowly. (See the diagram on page 190.)

Nail bed – *n-ay-l bed* – the area situated below the *nail plate*. It is made up of the *dermis* and has a pink appearance due to the *capillaries* in the dermis. (See the diagram on page 190.)

Nail brush – *n-ay-l br-ush* – an item of equipment used for removing grease and debris from the *nail plate*, ensuring nail enamel adheres (sticks) well.

Nail buffer – *n-ay-l buf-er* – an item of equipment used to smooth and polish the nails when nail enamel is not required.

Nail conditioner – *n-ay-l kon-di-sh-on-er* – a product used to strengthen and rebuild weak and damaged nails.

Nail enamel – *n-ay-l en-am-el* – a cosmetic lacquer applied to the finger and toe nails for decoration and protection. It is made from nitrocellulose (a flexible lacquer) dissolved in a *solvent* with coloured *pigments*. Also called nail polish or nail varnish.

Nail enamel remover – *n-ay-l en-am-el re-moo-ver* – a liquid *solvent* formulated to remove enamel from the *nail plate*. It contains *acetone* or ethyl acetate, which are commonly used solvents, as well as other ingredients to reduce the harmful effects of the solvent on the nail plate.

Nail form – *n-ay-l for-m* – a pre-moulded shape used to help create false nail extensions and which may be used instead of nail tips. Nail forms can be *(continued)*

117

disposable paper forms with a sticky back or reusable metal, plastic or Teflon-coated forms – these are shaped to fit any size of nail and must be *sterilised* after use.

Nail groove – *n-ay-l gr-oo-v* – a furrow at the side of a nail along which the *nail plate* moves as it grows. It acts as a guideline for the nail to follow. (See the diagram on page 190.)

Nail hardener – *n-ay-l har-den-er* – a product applied to the nail to increase the strength of the *nail plate*. It must not be used permanently as the nails may become brittle with constant use.

Nail plate – *n-ay-l pl-ay-t* – the visible portion of the nail which rests on the *nail bed* and ends in the *free edge*. It protects the ends of the fingers and toes and is made from the protein *keratin*. It is strong and flexible and made from many layers of dead, flattened *cells*. (See the diagram on page 190.)

Nail repair – *n-ay-l re-per* – a procedure used during a *manicure*, *pedicure* or in the maintenance of nail extensions. It

involves strengthening a break, split or tear in the *nail plate* using glue, a *fibreglass wrap*, a *silk wrap*, *gel* or acrylic.

Nail strengthener – *n-ay-l st-ren-g-th-en-er* – a base coat applied to the nail specifically to bond together the layers of the *nail plate* and make them more resistant to damage. Strengtheners may contain a combination of *resin*, *proteins*, conditioners and in some cases nylon fibres.

Nanospheres – *nan-os-f-eer-s* – microscopic delivery systems or lipids (fatty chemicals) made of water and fat, filled with active ingredients and used within *cosmetics* to transport substances deep into the skin.

Nasalis – *n-ay-sar-lis* – a small *muscle* covering the front of the nose. Its action is to compress (squeeze in) the nostrils. (See the diagram on page 192.)

Nasolabial folds – *nay-so-lab-ee-al f-old-s* – the creases that run from the sides of the nose to the sides of the mouth. As people age these become more prominent. They are caused by excess skin, thinning of the skin and drooping of cheek fat.

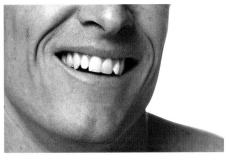

Nasolabial folds

National Occupational Standards – *n-ash-on-al ok-you-pay-sh-on-al st-and-ar-d-s* – statements of the skills, knowledge and understanding needed in a profession that clearly define the outcomes of competent performance.

Navicular bone – *nav-ik-you-lar b-oh-n* – one of the **tarsal bones** found in the foot.

Needs – *nee-d-s* – things that are required, desired or wanted.

Nephron – *ne-f-r-on* – the functional unit of the kidney that is responsible for purifying and filtering the blood.

Nerve – *n-er-v* – a bundle of fibres that conducts impulses (signals) to and from the brain or spinal cord (part of the **central nervous system** that runs up the spine and joins the brain) and the body. **Sensory nerves** are **afferent** nerves that carry information from the body to the brain and spinal cord. **Motor nerves** are **efferent** nerves that carry impulses away from the brain and spinal cord to the body.

Nerve plexus – *n-er-v pl-x-us* – a network of intersecting (criss-crossing) nerves.

Nervous system – *ner-v-us sis-t-em* – the body's control system. It collects, transmits (sends) and processes (sorts and deals with) information, then initiates the most appropriate response in order to maintain balance in the body. It is divided into the **central nervous system** and the **peripheral nervous system**. The central nervous system consists of the brain and spinal cord. It obtains information from the body and then sends out instructions in response. The peripheral nervous system is responsible for body functions that are not under conscious control, such as **digestion**. The peripheral nervous system is divided into the **somatic** *(continued)*

119

nervous system and the *autonomic nervous system*. The somatic system is associated with voluntary control of body movements. The autonomic system controls *homeostasis* and is divided into the *sympathetic nervous system* and the *parasympathetic nervous system*. (See the diagram on page 201.)

Neuralgia – *new-ral-ja* – a disorder characterised by pain that extends along the course of one or more nerves.

Neuritis – *new-r-eye-tis* – *inflammation* of a *nerve*.

Neuron – *new-ron* – a nerve cell.

Neutraliser – *new-tr-al-eye-s-er* – a substance mixed with or applied to another to make it ineffective or to counteract its activity.

Nodule – *nod-you-l* – a small mass of *tissue*, which is normally *benign* (harmless) and often painless.

Non-comedogenic – *non kom-e-doh-jen-ik* – indicates that a product will not block the *pores* in the skin.

Normal skin – *n-or-mal sk-in* – a balanced *skin type* with a clear complexion, even colour and smooth texture. Cell renewal and *exfoliation* of dead skin cells are working in harmony and the *sebaceous glands* produce sufficient natural oil to maintain a soft and supple skin. This skin type has a high degree of *elasticity* and efficient *collagen* production, contributing to the overall healthy appearance.

Nucleus – *new-k-lee-us* – part of a cell that contains *genetic* information – the hereditary (inherited) factors that control the cell's growth and reproduction. (See the diagram on page 188.) *Also* the central part of an *atom*, made up of *protons* and *neutrons*.

Nutrients – *new-tr-ee-en-t-s* – chemicals that provide nourishment and are essential to the body for growth, maintenance and repair. The nutrients needed by the human body are **proteins**, **carbohydrates**, fats, oils, minerals, **vitamins** and water.

Nutrition – *new-tri-sh-on* – the process by which a living organism obtains food and uses it for growth and repair. *Also* the study of **diet** and how this affects health.

Obesity – *oh-bee-sit-ee* – the excessive accumulation of fat in the body.

Objectives – *ob-jek-tiv-s* – goals to be achieved, desired outcomes or results.

Obliques – *oh-bl-ee-k-s* – *muscles* situated to the side and front of the *abdomen*. They comprise the internal and external obliques, with the external in front of the internal. They compress (squeeze) the *abdomen*, and help to *flex* and rotate the vertebral column (spine).

Occlusive – *ok-loo-siv* – creates an airtight and watertight barrier.

Oedema – *oh-dee-ma* – a build-up of excess fluid in the body leading to swelling of the *tissues*, most commonly in the ankles or legs. It occurs when the body's normal fluid balance is disturbed. It may be caused by heat, immobility (lack of movement), pregnancy, an increase in pressure within the *blood vessels*, a decrease in the amount of *proteins* in the blood or an underlying medical condition.

Oesophagus – *ee-sof-a-gus* – a muscular tube through which food travels from the mouth to the stomach. It is about 23 centimetres long and extends down from the *pharynx* immediately below the windpipe. It is lined with mucous *membrane*, which secretes (releases) a lubricating fluid. The muscular walls contract (tighten) to move the food along. This process is called *peristalsis*.

Oestrogen – *ees-tro-jen* – a *hormone* produced by the *ovaries* that controls female sexual development, promotes the growth of female secondary sexual characteristics at puberty (e.g. development of breasts), stimulates egg production and prepares the lining of the *uterus* for pregnancy.

Ohm – *oh-m* – a unit of electrical *resistance*.

Oil – *oy-l* – a lubricant (a substance that allows ease of movement) used in *massage* for its moisturising, nourishing and softening effects on the skin.

Oily skin – *oy-l-ee s-k-in* – a *skin type* characterised by a shiny appearance, thick *epidermis*, sallow colour, open *pores* and being prone to *comedones*. Caused by overactive *sebaceous glands*, it is more common in adolescent skins but can occur at any time.

Olfactory – *ol-fak-t-or-ee* – relating to the sense of smell.

Olfactory system – *ol-fak-t-or-ee sis-t-em* – the sensory (to do with the senses) system responsible for the sense of smell. It supplies us with valuable information about the environment and provides us with a warning system about dangerous smells (e.g. smoke or gas). It identifies odour, determines the concentration (strength) of an odour, distinguishes between different odours, recognises the same odour in different concentrations and matches the odour with memory.

Oligomer – *ol-ee-go-mer* – a chemical structure, consisting of a limited number of *monomers* bonded together. It is shorter than a *polymer*, which can be made of a limitless number of monomers.

Onychatrophia – *on-ee-cat-row-fee-a* – the wasting away of the *nail plate*, which becomes smaller and may fall off completely.

Onychauxis – *on-ee-kor-k-sis* – thickening of the *nail plate*. This may be the result of an internal disorder or of constant irritation, such as a badly fitting shoe.

Onychia – *on-nik-ee-a* – an *inflammation* occurring somewhere around or under the nail. There may also be swelling or the presence of pus. It may be caused by poor *hygiene* or infected manicure instruments.

Onychocryptosis – *on-ee-ko-k-rip-toe-sis* – this occurs when the *nail plate* grows into the flesh of the nail wall. It is most common on the big toe. The cause may be incorrect cutting and filing, pressure from ill-fitting shoes or neglect. Also known as an ingrown nail.

Onychogryphosis – *on-ee-ko-gr-eye-f-oh-sis* – an enlarged nail with an increased curve. *(continued)*

This is caused by an increase in the production of the horny cells (see **keratinisation**) of the **nail plate**, leading to curvature of the **free edge** which resembles a ram's horn. It is more common in older people and may be caused through neglect, age or ill-fitting shoes.

Onycholisis – *on-ee-ko-l-eye-sis* – a gradual separation of the **nail plate** from the **nail bed** when the nail loosens but does not come away completely. It may be caused by **eczema** or **psoriasis** on the nail bed, internal disorders or rough treatment such as poking a sharp object under the **free edge**.

Onychomadesis – *on-ee-ko-mad-ee-sis* – complete loss of nails.

Onychomalacia – *on-ee-ko-mal-ay-sh-a* – soft nails.

Onychomycosis – *on-ee-ko-mee-ko-sis* – a fungal **infection** of the nails, usually resulting from the spread of a fungal infection of the skin. It is normally painless and may be ignored for years. The nail progressively changes in colour and quality and all layers of the **nail plate**, beneath and on top, are affected. Also known as tinea unguium.

Onychophagy – *on-ee-ko-f-a-j-ee* – a technical term for bitten nails and in some cases bitten **cuticles** around the nails. Nail biting is a nervous habit, which eventually exposes the **hyponychium** and causes very weak or deformed nails. The only cure is to stop biting the nails, but regular **manicures** with moisturising treatments will greatly improve the condition.

Onychophyma – *on-ee-ko-fee-ma* – painful swelling of the nails.

Onychoptosis – *on-ee-kop-toe-sis* – periodic shedding of part or all of the nail.

Onychorrhexis – *on-ee-ko-rex-is* – dry, brittle nails which split or peel.

Onychosis – *on-ee-k-oh-sis* – any disease or disorder of the nail.

Onychotillomania – *on-ee-ko-till-oh-may-nee-a* – compulsive picking at the nail.

Orange flower water – *o-ran-j fl-ow-er w-or-t-er* – a natural extract made by distilling (extracting a substance from) orange blossoms which is used as a skin *toning lotion*.

Orange stick – *o-ran-j st-ik* – a thin wooden tool used in *manicure* to push back the *cuticles* and to remove small amounts of product from *applicators* to apply to the nail or cuticle.

Orbicularis oculi – *or-bik-you-lar-is ok-you-l-eye* – a *sphincter* muscle that surrounds the eye orbit and extends out to the temple and cheek. It closes the eyelid and compresses (squeezes) the lacrimal (tear) gland, aiding the flow of tears over the eye. (See the diagram on page 192.)

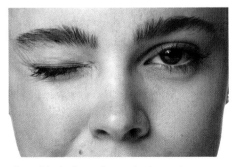

The orbicularis oculi muscle closes the eye

Orbicularis oris – *or-bik you-l-ar-is or-is* – a *sphincter* muscle around the mouth, the action of which is to pucker the lips, as in kissing. (See the diagram on page 192.)

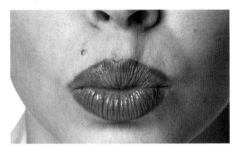

The orbicularis oris muscle puckers the lips

Organisational requirements – *or-gan-eyes-ay-shon-al re-kw-eye-r-men-t-s* – beauty therapy procedures, rules and regulations issued by the salon management.

Origin – *o-ri-jin* – the fixed attachment of a *muscle* to a bone, i.e. the end of the muscle attached to the bone that remains relatively still during muscle *contraction*. *Also* where something or someone comes from.

Osmoregulation – *os-m-oh-reg-you-lay-shon* – the body's method of controlling the levels of water and mineral salts in the blood.

Osmosis – *os-m-oh-sis* – the passage of dissolved substances through a semi-permeable (allows only some substances through) **membrane**.

Ossification – *oss-if-ik-ay-shon* – the process of bone formation.

Osteoblast – *os-tee-oh-blas-t* – a **cell** that makes bone.

Osteoclast – *os-tee-oh-k-las-t* – a **cell** that breaks down bone, and absorbs and removes unwanted **tissue**.

Osteocyte – *os-tee-oh-s-eye-t* – a mature bone **cell**, which maintains bone as living **tissue**.

Osteoporosis – *os-tee-oh-p-or-oh-sis* – a disease that causes the bones to become fragile and more likely to break. It can progress painlessly and only become evident when a bone breaks. It is common in post-menopausal (who have been through the **menopause**) women.

Outcomes – *ow-t-kum-s* – results of effort, goals attained or tasks completed.

Outer root sheath – *ow-t-er roo-t sh-ee-th* – the layer situated between the **inner root sheath** and the **connective tissue** sheath of the **hair follicle**. It varies in thickness depending on the size of the follicle. (See the diagram on page 190.)

Ovary – *oh-va-ree* – the female sexual **gland**. There are two ovaries, one on each side of the **pelvic girdle**. The ovaries are both **exocrine** and **endocrine glands** They are egg-producing reproductive organs (exocrine function) and also secrete (release) the **hormones oestrogen** and **progesterone** (endocrine function). (See the diagram on page 200.)

Overheads – *oh-v-er-hed-s* – the operating expenses of running a business, including: rent, rates, heating, lighting, laundry, telephone, wages, equipment, products and consumables.

Overlay – *oh-ver-lay* – see **wrap**.

Overtrading – *oh-ver tr-ay-din-g* – the situation of a business when it spends more cash than it has coming in.

Oxidisation – *ox-ee-d-eye-say-sh-on* – the combination of a substance with oxygen, causing the loss of *electrons* from *atoms* in the substance. The process of oxidisation causes *free radical* damage in the body, which contributes to premature (early) ageing through cellular degeneration (damage to the *cells*). *Antioxidants*, in particular *vitamins* A, C and E, help counteract the oxidisation process. (An example of oxidisation is when a cut apple turns brown on exposure to air.) Also known as oxidative stress.

Oxygen – *oks-ee-jen* – a colourless, odourless, tasteless gas, essential in the *respiration* of all animals and plants.

Oxygenated blood – *ox-ij-en-ay-ted b-l-ud* – blood that has high levels of *oxygen*. (See the diagram on page 198.)

Oxytocin – *ok-see-toe-sin* – a *hormone* produced by the *posterior* lobe (section) of the *pituitary gland*. It stimulates the *contraction* of the *smooth muscle* of the *uterus* in order to deliver the foetus (unborn baby) and stimulates milk flow after the birth.

Ozone – *oh-z-oh-n* – condensed *oxygen*; a *molecule* consisting of three oxygen *atoms* formed by electrical discharges in the air. It is found in large amounts in the upper layers of the earth's atmosphere. It is a powerful oxidant (causes *oxidisation*) and is therefore damaging to cell structure. It has a characteristic odour and is used as a disinfectant. It is produced in direct high-frequency treatments when the *high-frequency current* mixes with oxygen.

Painting techniques – *p-ay-n-tin-g tek-n-ee-k-s* – a range of nail art methods which can include freehand, brushes, textured sponges, colour shapers and marbling techniques.

Pancreas – *pan-k-ree-as* – an organ in the **abdomen**, that is part of both the **digestive system** and the **endocrine system**. It is an **exocrine gland**, secreting (releasing) pancreatic (from the pancreas) juice that contains digestive **enzymes** to break down food. It is also an **endocrine gland**, secreting **hormones** to regulate **blood glucose** levels. (See the diagram on page 200.)

Papilla – *pap-il-a* – a small projection (bulge) in the skin between the **epidermis** and **dermis** at the base of the **hair follicle**. (See the diagram on page 190.)

Papillary layer – *pap-il-a-ree lay-er* – the upper part of the **dermis** just beneath the **epidermis**. (See the diagram on page 189.)

Papule – *pap-you-l* – a small, solid, round bump in the skin, which does not contain pus.

Papules often occur in clusters and may be caused by **inflammation**, **infection**, **abrasion**, accumulated (built up) skin **secretions** or **hyperkeratinisation**. They may in some cases be transitional (changing from one state to another) **lesions** that later become **vesicles** or **pustules**.

Paraffin wax – *pa-ra-fin w-ak-s* – a white substance, with no taste or smell and with a melting point of 47– 64°C. Used in face, hand, foot and body masks to transfer heat to the **tissues** and to soften the skin, soothe **muscles**, induce perspiration (sweating) and exfoliate dead skin cells.

Parasite – *pa-ra-s-eye-t* – an organism that lives on or in another organism from which it receives nourishment.

Parasitic infection – *pa-ra-sit-ik in-fek-sh-on* – disease caused by a **parasite** present in the body.

Parasympathetic nervous system – *pa-ra-sim-pa-th-et-ik ner-vus-sis-tem* – the part of the **autonomic nervous system** that is responsible for such things as slowing the heart, constricting (narrowing) the pupils, dilating (widening) *blood vessels* and stimulating the *digestive system*, *reproductive system* and *urinary system*.

Parathormone – *pa-ra-th-or-m-oh-n* – a *hormone* secreted (released) by the *parathyroid glands* which is critical to the blance of calcium and phosphorus in the body. It increases calcium in the blood by releasing it from the bones when required. Also known as parathyroid hormone.

Parathyroid glands – *pa-ra-th-eye-r-oy-d gl-and-s* – four small *endocrine gland*s in the neck, usually located behind the *thyroid gland*. The purpose of these glands is to regulate the calcium level in the body so that the *nervous system* and the *muscular system* can function efficiently. (See the diagram on page 200.)

Parental consent – *p-ar-en-t-al kon-sen-t* – permission given by a parent for a child to have a *treatment* or service.

Paronychia – *pa-r-oh-nik-ee-ah* – an *infection* at the side or base of a nail caused by *bacteria* entering the skin through a crack or tear in the *tissue* around the nail. It is characterised by pain, redness and swelling. Also known as a *whitlow*.

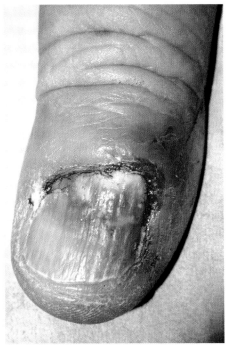

Paronychia

Partnership – *par-t-ner-sh-ip* – the legal form a business takes when two or more people (the partners) provide the start-up cash and share the risks, costs, reponsibilities and workload in the business. Each partner *(continued)* is liable for the debts of the others, so it is advisable to draw up a legal partnership agreement.

Pathogenic – *pa-th-oh-jen-ik* – harmful and disease-producing.

Payment – *pay-men-t* – the act of paying.

Payment cards – *pay-men-t k-ar-d-s* – *debit* or *credit cards* used instead of cash to pay for goods and services.

Pectorals – *pek-tor-al-s* – two pairs of *muscles* forming the front of the upper chest wall: the pectoralis major and minor. They pull the upper arms towards or across the chest.

Pedicure – *ped-ik-y-or* – a *treatment* of the feet that improves the appearance of the feet and toe nails. It helps to prevent nail diseases and disorders. A pedicure includes cleansing, hard skin removal, nail filing, *cuticle* treatment, foot and leg *massage* and nail enamel application. Sometimes, additional treatments to nourish or hydrate the skin will be included in the form of a mask or *thermal* treatment.

Pelvic girdle – *pel-vik g-er-d-l* – a group of bones that connects the torso and the legs, supports and balances the torso, and contains and supports the intestines, urinary bladder and internal sex organs. It consists of two hip bones connected in front at the pubic symphysis (the join where the two pubic bones meet) and behind by the sacrum (triangular-shaped bone between the fifth lumbar *vertebra* and the coccyx). Each hip bone is made up of the ilium, ischium and pubis. (See the diagram on page 195.)

Percussion – *per-ku-sh-on* – *massage* manipulations using rapid stimulating movements of the hands, including *hacking*, *clapping*, beating and pounding. Percussion movements are adapted for facial massage by using the palmar (front) surfaces of the fingertips to perform digital (with the fingers) hacking and tapping. Also known as tapotement.

Percussion vibrator – *per-ku-sh-on v-eye-br-ay-tor* – a mechanical, hand-held massager, used on small areas of the body. It has small, detachable heads to provide different effects.

Perform – *per-for-m* – to carry out a work function to the specified standard.

Performance – *per-for-man-s* – the carrying out of work and the way in which it is achieved.

Perfume – *per-f-you-m* – a pleasant-smelling liquid – often a mixture of *essential oils*, aroma compounds (chemical *fragrance*), stabilising agents, *preservatives* and *solvent*. Perfume is applied to the body for its fragrance, or used in other ways such as added to soaps, air fresheners, pot pourri, scented candles, bath products and skin care ranges.

Peripheral nervous system – *pe-ri-fe-ral ner-vus sis-tem* – the part of the *nervous system* that consists of *nerves* and *neurons* and is divided into the *somatic nervous system* and the *autonomic nervous system*.

Peristalsis – *pe-ris-tal-sis* – a pattern of *smooth muscle* contractions in the digestive tract (consisting of the *oesophagus*, stomach and small and large intestines) that propels food through the *digestive system*. The *contraction* of smooth, circular muscles prevents food moving backwards, while the contraction of longitudinal (running along the length) muscle pushes the food forward through the digestive tract.

Perm – *p-er-m* – to permanently curl the hair or eyelashes.

Perm lotion – *p-er-m l-oh-sh-on* – an *alkaline* substance applied to the hair as part of the *perming* process. It reacts with the *keratin* in the *cortex* of the hair to break down the *disulphide bonds* within and between the *protein* chains in the hair. The hair then swells and softens so that it can stretch to take the shape of hair curlers or eyelash rods.

Permeable – *per-mee-a-b-l* – allows liquids or gases to pass through.

Perionychium – *pe-r-ee-on-ik-ee-um* – the *cuticle* at the sides of the *nail plate*. It is the site of *hangnails*, ingrown nails (*onychocryptosis*) and the infection *paronychia*. (See the diagram on page 190.) Also known as the *paronychial edge*.

Person specification – *p-er-son spe-si-fi-k-ay-sh-on* – a list of the qualities, skills, knowledge and experience required in job applicants. These should be categorised as essential and desirable to help the interviewer make the right choice of applicant for the job.

Personal appearance – *p-er-son-al ap-ee-r-an-s* – how an individual looks, including the condition and style of their hair and clothes, their *posture*, facial expression and makeup, etc. *Also* the act of a person coming into view or making a visit.

Personal data – *p-er-son-al d-ay-t-a* – information about a person, which allows the person to be identified.

Personal development – *p-er-son-al de-vel-op-men-t* – an individual's growth, progression and improvement.

Personal presentation – *p-er-son-al pr-es-en-t-ay-sh-on* – the manner, style and appearance of an individual to suit a particular environment or occasion. A *beauty therapist* must always look professional, wearing the correct uniform that is clean and

crease-free, appropriate shoes, a minimum amount of jewellery conforming to company policy, with hair tidy and off the face, short clean nails free from nail enamel, suitable makeup and fragrance and, when necessary, the correct personal protective equipment.

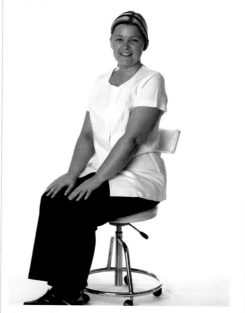

Personal presentation is very important for a professional beauty therapist

Personal safety – *p-er-son-al say-f-tee* – an individual's responsibility to make sure they are free from danger of harm or injury and not taking unnecessary risks.

Petrissage – *pet-ri-s-ar-j* – deep *massage* movements with applied pressure to compress the underlying muscles. *Kneading*, *wringing*, *picking up*, *frictions* and *skin rolling* are all petrissage movements performed with the padded palmar (front) surfaces of the hands, fingers and thumbs. The hands should be moulded to the area and the movements should be slow and rhythmical.

Petroleum jelly – *pet-r-oh-lee-um je-lee* – a semi-solid waxy substance with no smell or taste. When applied to the skin it acts as an *occlusive*, sealing the skin, repelling water and preventing evaporation of moisture. In *eyelash and eyebrow tinting* it is used to protect the skin from staining.

pH – the degree of *alkalinity* and *acidity* in a substance measured on a scale ranging from 0 (strongly acid) to 14.0 (strongly alkaline), with 7.0 being neutral. The pH of the skin is 4.0–5.5 and the eyes have a pH of 7.4–7.6.

Phagocyte – *fag-oh-s-eye-t* – a *cell* transported in the blood that ingests (consumes) and destroys foreign matter in a process known as phagocytosis.

Phalanges – *fa-lan-jee-s* – the bones of the fingers or toes. (See the diagram on page 197.)

Pharynx – *fa-rin-x* – the passage from the mouth to the larynx (voicebox) and *oesophagus*, through which air passes.

Phlebitis – *fl-ee-by-t-is* – *inflammation* of a superficial (on or near the surface) or deep *vein*. Superficial phlebitis affects veins on the surface of the skin; deep vein thrombophlebitis affects the larger vessels deep in the legs. Phlebitis can be caused by a complication following a medical or surgical procedure, prolonged inactivity, *varicose veins*, *obesity*, smoking or an injury.

Photo-ageing – *f-oh-toe ay-jin-g* – a series of changes in the skin as a result of sun exposure or *ultraviolet radiation*.

Photo rejuvenation – *f-oh-toe-ree-joo-ven-ay-shon* – treatment using *laser* light to smooth skin, reduce *wrinkles*, *age spots*, broken *capillaries* and *rosacea*.

Photosensitise – *f-oh-toe-sen-sit-eye-s* – to make sensitive and react badly to **ultraviolet light**.

Photosensitiser – *f-oh-toe-sen-sit-eyes-er* – an ingredient that can cause the skin to become irritated or inflamed when exposed to sunlight.

Photosensitivity – *f-oh-toe-sen-sit-iv-it-ee* – a reaction to sunlight, real or artificial, that produces a **rash** on the skin. It may be caused by exposure to **ultraviolet radiation**, topical (applied to the skin) application of a product that reacts with ultraviolet light, a metabolic defect (see **metabolism**), a **genetic** disorder or a pre-existing skin disease. Also known as photodermatosis.

Physical – *fiz-ik-al* – relating to the body and its features.

Physical effects – *fiz-ik-al ef-x* – reactions to a stimulus (something that causes a reaction) that may be seen externally, such as a change in skin colour or texture after a facial.

Physiological effects – *fiz-ee-oh-loj-ik-al ef-x* – reactions to a stimulus that occur within the body, affecting any of the body's systems. For example, an increase in circulation or flow of **lymph** during massage.

Physiology – *fiz-ee-ol-o-jee* – the biological study of the functions of living organisms: how all the different parts of the organism work, what they do and how they interact with each other.

Phytotherapy – *f-eye-t-oh-th-e-rap-ee* – the use in **therapy** of plants, herbs, seaweed, **essential oils** and botanical (from plants) extracts, together with **massage**, **body wraps**, packs, water, steam and inhalation (breathing in).

Picking up – *pik-in-g up* – a **kneading** massage manipulation that can be performed single-handed or double-handed. The technique is to lift, squeeze and relax the muscle being massaged and the effects are to stimulate circulation and **lymph** flow, release tension and relax muscles.

Pigment – *pig-men-t* – a colouring matter or substance that may be naturally occurring, such as **melanin** in the skin, or added to **cosmetics** to provide different colours.

Pili multigemini – *p-eye-l-eye mul-tee-jem-in-eye* – a **hair follicle** with several **hair shafts**, each formed by a single branch of **dermal papilla**, which is surrounded by all layers present in a normal follicle except for the **outer root sheath** cells. Instead, the outer root sheath surrounds the entire follicle. Also known as a compound follicle.

Pilosebaceous unit – *p-eye-loh-seb-ay-sh-us y-oo-n-it* – consists of the **hair shaft**, **hair follicle**, the **sebaceous gland** and the **arrector pili muscle**. (See the diagram on page 190.)

Pineal gland – *p-eye-nee-al gl-and* – a small **endocrine gland** situated in the brain, responsible for the production and release of **melatonin**. It is stimulated by darkness and inhibited (slowed down) by light. (See the diagram on page 200.) Also called the epiphysis.

Piriformis – *pi-ri-for-mis* – a small narrow **muscle** of the hip situated deep in the buttocks that rotates the leg outwards. It runs

from the base of the spine to the **femur**.

Pitting – *pit-in-g* – small, indented scars that result from over-treatment of the **hair follicle** during **electrical epilation**. They will improve in time, depending on the level of damage caused. Pitting also occurs in the **nail plate** when the **nail be**d beneath is affected by psoriasis.

Pituitary gland – *pit-you-it-a-ree gl-and* – sometimes known as the 'master' gland of the **endocrine system** because it controls the function of the other **endocrine glands**. It is situated at the base of the brain and is attached to the **hypothalamus** by **nerve** fibres. It consists of two lobes (sections): **anterior** and **posterior**. The anterior lobe secretes (releases): **somatotrophin**, **adrenocorticotrophic hormone** (ACTH), thyroid stimulating hormone (TSH), **follicle stimulating hormone** (FSH), **luteinising hormone** (LH) and **prolactin** (PRL). The posterior lobe secretes: **antidiuretic hormone** (ADH) and **oxytocin**. **Melanocyte stimulating hormone** (MSH) is secreted by an intermediate lobe, which is a thin layer of *(continued)* cells between the anterior and posterior lobes. The pituitary gland controls growth, **blood pressure**, some aspects of pregnancy and birth, lactation (milk production), sex organ function, **thyroid** function, **metabolism** and water regulation. (See the diagram on page 200.)

Plan – pl-an – a scheme or method worked out in advance to achieve set **objectives**.

Planning permission – pl-an-in-g per-mi-shon – a procedure that a business has to go through if it wants to build new premises or change the use of or extend an existing building. An application has to be made to the local planning department asking for consent to do the building work.

Plant room – pl-an-t r-oo-m – the room near a swimming pool or spa that contains the filtration (the process of removing solid particles from water) and chemical dosing systems and stores the chemicals used to treat the water and keep it clean, all of which are essential requirements in maintaining health and safety in the spa.

Plantar – pl-ant-ar – on the sole of the foot.

Plantarflexion – pl-ant-ar-flek-shon – a movement that increases the angle between the foot and ankle, when the toes are pointed downwards.

Plasma – pl-as-ma – the yellowish, liquid part of blood, in which cells are suspended (hanging). It makes up to 50 per cent of the total volume of the blood and contains vital **proteins**, including: fibrinogen, which helps with blood clotting; globulins such as **haemoglobin** to help transport oxygen; and serum albumin (which helps body fluid move into body tissues). Plasma is a means of transport for **glucose**, lipids (fatty chemicals), **amino acids**, **hormones**, the end products of **metabolism**, **carbon dioxide** and **oxygen**.

Plasticiser – pl-as-tis-eyes-er – an ingredient in a cosmetic preparation such as **nail enamel**, which is included to add viscosity (thickness), flexibility and pliability (easily bent without breaking).

Platelets – pl-ay-t-lets – irregularly shaped, colourless particles present in blood, which aid clotting and therefore reduce blood loss.

Platysma – *pl-at-is-ma* – a thin sheet of *muscle* positioned between the *clavicle* and the jaw, the action of which is to pull down the jaw and lower lip. (See the diagram on page 192.)

Plucking – *pl-uk-in-g* – forcibly removing hair from the *hair follicle* using *tweezers*. Also known as tweezing.

Polarity switch – *po-la-rit-ee sw-i-t-ch* – a device on a *galvanic unit* which allows the polarity (the use of either positive or negative electrical charges) to be changed from positive to negative.

Policy – *pol-is-ee* – a plan, principle or procedure that has been decided and which is used to influence and determine decisions, actions and other matters.

Polish secures – *po-li-sh sek-your-s* – jewellery for the nails used in nail art. They are small stones which are secured in place by applying them to the nail plate between a layer of enamel and a top coat.

Polycystic ovarian syndrome (PCOS) – *pol-ee-sis-tik oh-ver-ee-an sin-dr-oh-m* – a condition associated with multiple *cysts* in the ovaries. Symptoms include irregular periods, excess hair growth, *acne* and *obesity*. It is thought that sufferers have a *genetic* predisposition (tendency) to this condition, but increased production of *androgens* and *oestrogen*, together with an increased resistance to *insulin*, cause the syndrome. Also known as Stein-Leventhal syndrome.

Polymer – *pol-i-m-er* – a large *molecule* made up of smaller molecules or *monomers*, connected by chemical bonds.

Polymerisation – *pol-im-er-eye-say-sh-on* – the chemical process that occurs when acrylic components, liquid and powder mix together and activate to form a solid mass used to make an *acrylic nail*.

Pore – *p-or* – a minute opening in the skin which allows *sweat* to be excreted (eliminated). (See the diagram on page 189.)

Port wine stain – *p-or-t w-eye-n st-ay-n* – a red or purple, irregular-shaped area of skin, present from birth. It develops in areas lacking small *nerves* that control the ability of small *blood vessels* to constrict (become narrower). As a result the blood vessels stay open all the time and this shows up as permanent colour. It may be treated by *laser* or *cosmetic camouflage*.

Post-inflammatory hyperpigmentation – *p-oh-st in-fl-am-at-or-ee h-eye-per-pig-men-t-ay-sh-on* – discoloration (change from the normal colour) of the skin after a skin disease or disorder has healed, e.g. *acne vulgaris*, *allergies*, injury, *eczema* or burns. The areas affected can be light brown to black in colour and they may become darker when exposed to sunlight. They are more common in darker skins. The colour will return to normal over time. See also *hyperpigmentation*.

Posterior – *pos-tee-ree-or* – on or at the back. *Also* behind.

Posture – *pos-t-y-or* – the position of the human body when standing, sitting or lying down. Good posture keeps the bones

and *joints* in the correct alignment so that *muscles* are being used properly and it contributes to a good appearance. Also a person's attitude or bearing.

Potential – *p-oh-ten-sh-al* – having the qualities or ability to develop and lead to future success.

Potentiometer – *poh-ten-she-om-e-ter* – an electrical device that varies the voltage in an electrical circuit.

Powder – *pow-der* – an ingredient used in clay *face masks*, *cosmetics*, as a massage medium and in nail products.

Pre-blended – *pr-ee-blen-d-ed* – a number of ingredients mixed smoothly together in advance of their use.

Predisposition test – *pr-ee-dis-poh-si-shon te-st* – a procedure carried out to assess if there might be an adverse reaction to the application of a specific substance. A small amount of the substance is placed on the skin to test for an *allergic* response. A negative reaction means the treatment may proceed. A client must have a predisposition test before an eyelash tint or perm.

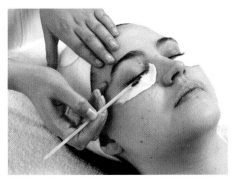

A predisposition test must be carried out before an eyelash tint

Premises – *pr-em-is-es* – a building or part of a building and the land belonging to it occupied by a business.

Preparation – *prep-a-ray-shon* – a process before an activity to ensure that everything is ready to meet the **objectives**.

Prepare – *pr-e-p-air* – to assemble required items in advance, to put in proper order or to make oneself ready for an activity.

Presentation – *pre-zen-tay-sh-on* – a demonstration, lecture, speech, exhibition or performance.

Preservative – *pre-ser-va-tiv* – an ingredient in cosmetics that prevents contamination caused by **bacteria**.

Prickle cell layer – *prik-l sel lay-er* – see **stratum spinosum**.

Procerus – *pro-ser-us* – a small facial **muscle** situated over the nasal bone near the eyebrows. Its action is to depress (pull down) the eyebrow and cause horizontal wrinkles on the bridge of the nose. (See the diagram on page 192.)

Process payment – *pr-oh-s-es p-ay-men-t* – to accept **cash**, **cheques**, **credit** and **debit cards**, gift vouchers and other **cash equivalents** in return for goods and services. The procedure includes providing an itemised bill, accepting payment, making security checks and issuing a receipt.

Product knowledge – *prod-uk-t n-o-led-j* – all the information relating to the goods used to provide treatments and the commodities offered for sale that the therapist needs to have. Product knowledge includes the **features**, **benefits** and *(continued)*

unique selling points of the products, and should enable the therapist to provide accurate and detailed information to a client when making a sale.

Product liability insurance – *prod-uk-t l-eye-a-bil-it-ee in-sh-or-an-s* – a type of financial cover to protect a business if a client seeks compensation from being injured or harmed by defective products.

Productivity – *prod-uk-tiv-it-ee* – the amount of work achieved in a given time, a measure of worker efficiency.

Professional indemnity insurance – *pro-fes-sh-on-l in-dem-nit-ee in-sh-or-an-s* – a type of financial cover to protect against the risks involved in doing a job. It protects the business against compensation sought by a client if mistakes have been made or if negligence (carelessness) is proved.

Progesterone – *pr-o-jest-er-oh-n* – a *hormone* secreted (released) by the *ovaries* in the second two weeks of the *menstrual cycle*. It is essential for building and maintaining the

lining of the *uterus* ready to receive a fertilised egg.

Prolactin – *pr-oh-lak-tin* – a *hormone* secreted by the *anterior* lobe (section) of the *pituitary gland*. It stimulates lactation (milk production).

Promote – *pr-o-m-oh-t* – to encourage sales through publicity or advertising. *Also* to give a person a higher-level position in an organisation.

Promotion – *pr-o-m-oh-shon* – a special offer, an activity or product designed to advertise or publicise an event, products, a cause or a business. It may include word of mouth, posters, an advertisement, personal appearance, demonstration, a newspaper article or a radio or TV commercial. *Also* the act of being given a higher-level position in an organisation.

Pronation – *pr-oh-nay-shon* – rotation of the hand or forearm so that the palm faces down or back.

Prone – *pr-oh-n* – lying face down.

Protein – p-r-oh-teen – organic (found in living tissue) *molecules* that contain carbon, hydrogen, *oxygen*, nitrogen and sulphur. Protein is a component of all living *cells* and forms the basis of living *tissue*. It is essential to have protein in the *diet* for growth and repair.

Provide – pr-o-v-eye-d – to supply, give or make available for use.

Proximal – prox-im-al – nearest to the point of origin or the *midline* of the body.

Pseudofolliculitis barbae – soo-doh-fol-ik-you-l-eye-tis bar-b-eye – a common condition of the beard area in Afro-Caribbean men and others with curly hair. It occurs when highly curved hairs grow back into the skin, causing *inflammation*. Over time this may cause a type of *keloid* scarring, which has the appearance of small hard bumps in the skin. Also known as shaving rash or razor bumps.

Pseudomonas aeruginosa – soo-do-m-oh-n-as er-rug-in-oh-sa – a flagellated (having long, thread-like extensions of cells to help it move) *bacterium* that thrives in moist environments, such as a spa or pool area. It is able to grow in temperatures up to 42°C and causes a number of *infections*.

Psoriasis – s-or-eye-sis – a common, chronic, inflammatory skin disorder characterised by raised, red patches of skin covered with silvery scales. It is an acceleration (speeding up) of the usual replacement process of the skin. It may occur on any part of the body, although common sites are elbows, knees and scalp. The cause is unknown, but the condition runs in families and a trigger such as a throat infection, injury, certain drugs and physical and emotional *stress* may cause it to appear.

Psychological – s-eye-ko-loj-ik-al – relating to the mind, mental state and emotions.

Psychological effect – s-eye-ko-loj-ik-al ef-ect – a reaction of the mind to a stimulus, which alters mood and feelings.

Pterygium – t-er-ij-ee-um – a forward growth of hardened *cuticle* over the *nail plate*.

Puberty – *p-you-ber-tee* – the first stage of adolescence when sexual maturity starts to become evident. It takes place in females between the ages of 11 and 14 and in males between the ages of 13 and 16. It is a time of physical and emotional changes, which are brought about by a huge increase in *hormones*: *oestrogen* in girls and *testosterone* in boys.

Public liability insurance – *pub-lik l-eye-a bil-it ee in-sh-or-an-s* – a type of financial cover for any compensation that a member of the public may be awarded as a result of injury or damage to them or their property caused by a business.

Pulmonary circulation – *pul-m-oh-na-ree ser-q-lay-sh-on* – the movement of *deoxygenated blood* from the heart to the lungs and the return of *oxygenated blood* to the heart. (See the diagram on page 198.)

Pulse – *pul-s* – a wave of pressure that passes along the arteries, indicating the pumping action of the heart. Also a short burst of energy.

Pumice stone – *pu-mis st-oh-n* – a lightweight volcanic stone used to remove hard skin, particularly on the feet.

Pustule – *pus-t-you-l* – an infected *papule* with a red, inflamed surrounding area and a yellow centre that develops at the opening of a *hair follicle* or *sweat gland* in the skin. The pus in the centre is formed by a combination of *bacteria* and a build-up of epidermal (skin) cells, together with infection-fighting *white blood cells*.

Quadriceps – *kw-od-ri-seps* – four extensor *muscles* (muscles that extend or straighten a limb) situated in the thigh: rectus femoris, vastus lateralis, vastus intermedius and vastus medialis. They *extend* the knee *joint* and are crucial in walking, running, jumping and squatting. The rectus femoris also *flexes* the hip.

Quaternary ammonium compound – *kw-or-ter-na-ree am-oh-nee-um kom-pow-n-d-s* – a highly potent (powerful) disinfectant with germicidal (kills germs) properties for *sanitising* instruments and work surfaces.

Questions – *kw-es-t-yons* – requests for information. Types of question include: open questions, closed questions and probing questions. Open questions are likely to receive a long answer, as they ask the person answering to think and reflect before they provide a detailed answer. Open questions begin with words such as what, why, how, when or describe. Closed questions can be answered with yes or no. They provide facts and are easy and quick to answer. Closed questions usually begin with words such as do, would, will, are, if. Probing questions are used when more detail is required, when answers are vague, when clarification is needed or if insufficient information has been provided.

Quick dry – *kwik dr-eye* – a special liquid formulation applied as a final coat over the top coat of enamel in a *manicure* or *pedicure* to speed up the drying time.

Radiation – *ray-dee-ay-shon* – waves of energy in the *electromagnetic spectrum* – a form of energy transmission that requires no conductive medium (a material that energy travels along, e.g. electric current down a wire) and so the energy travels through the air.

Radiotherapy – *ray-dee-oh-ther-ap-ee* – treatment of disease by means of x-rays or radioactive substances. Radiotherapy is a *contraindication* to many beauty treatments.

Radius – *ray-dee-us* – the bone of the forearm on the side of the thumb. (See the diagram on page 197.)

Rash – *ra-sh* – an eruption on the skin, characterised by redness, small *papules* and *vesicles*, that occurs as a result of contact with an external irritant, an illness or disease.

Rasul – *ras-ool* – a popular *spa* treatment. It is a deep-cleansing ritual of ancient origins, using micronised (finely ground) mud from Morocco that contains essential minerals such as silicon, magnesium, iron, calcium, potassium and sodium. The spa treatment combines steam, heat and water therapy with the application of mud. The rasul chamber is a steam room tiled and domed with a North African colour scheme of burnt orange and blue. Steam infused with herbs such as lemongrass, chamomile and lavender fills the chamber, benefiting the skin and the *respiratory system* and aiding *detoxification* of the body. There are usually several differently coloured muds that may be applied to the body and rubbed in while the *heat treatment* is being enjoyed. After a certain length of time a warm shower falls from the roof of the dome to gently wash away the mud.

Reception – *re-sep-shon* – an area in a salon, at or near the entrance, set aside for greeting clients, as a waiting area and for taking payment. The reception is also an ideal retail and display area. It provides the first impression of the salon and it should reflect the salon image, be inviting and put the client or visitor at ease.

Receptionist – *re-sep-shon-is-t* – a person employed to welcome and assist visitors to a business. The receptionist's duties include answering the telephone, booking appointments, welcoming clients and visitors, dealing with problems, *processing payments* and often *promoting* retail sales.

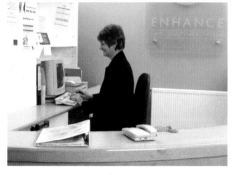

A receptionist at work

Record cards – *re-k-or-d k-ar-d-s* – a method of storing relevant information and *data* about clients.

Records – *re-k-or-d-s* – information or *data* collected and recorded in written format or in a *computer*.

Rectifier – *rek-t-if-eye-er* – an electrical device that converts *alternating current* to *direct current*.

Rectus abdominis – *rek-t-us ab-dom-in-is* – a large *muscle* of the *anterior* abdominal wall, which is divided into two parts on either side of the linea alba (a thin line of *connective tissue*). It *flexes* the vertebral column (spine) and draws the chest down. Also known as the six pack.

Reflexology – *ree-flex-ol-o-jee* – a *therapy* using ancient Chinese techniques. Specific points on the feet, hands or ears are stimulated to restore the flow of energy through the body and stimulate the body's self-healing processes. It reduces *stress*, promotes relaxation, improves circulation, revitalises and contributes to *homeostasis*.

Refund – *ree-fun-d* – to make a repayment of the cost of a purchase.

Regrowth – *ree-gr-oh-th* – hair that grows back after *depilation* or *electrical epilation* has been carried out.

Regulations – *reg-you-lay-shon-s* – principles, rules or laws that are intended to direct and influence behaviour and other activities.

Relevant person – *re-lev-ant* – the most appropriate individual.

Repair – *re-pair* – to strengthen, mend or restore to a good condition.

Reproductive system – *r-ee-pr-oh-duk-tiv sis-t-m* – a group of organs, **glands** and **hormones** in the male and female that contribute to the creation of a new life. The female reproductive system consists of **ovaries**, ova (eggs), **fallopian tubes**, **uterus**, cervix (lower part of the uterus where it joins the vagina), **endometrium** and vagina. The male reproductive system consists of urethra (passage for sperm, as well as urine), **glands**, scrotum (pouch containing the testes), **testes**, spermatozoa (sperm cells), vas deferens (carries sperm from the testes) and penis.

Resin – *re-s-in* – a viscous (thick) fluid that is secreted naturally by trees and is used in varnishes, adhesives, depilatory (removes hair) **wax**, **essential oil**, incense and **perfume**. Some resins are extracted for their **fragrance** and are used in essential oil blends.

Resin activator – *re-sin ak-tiv-ay-tor* – a substance that sets the glue when applying false nail extensions, to make it strong and non-porous (not able to absorb fluid).

Resin glue – *re-sin gl-oo* – an adhesive used to fix a nail extension or fabric **wrap** to the natural nail.

Resistance – *re-sis-tan-s* – opposition to something. Electrical resistance is opposition to the flow of current and is measured in **ohms**.

Resistor – *re-is-tor* – an electrical device to reduce current flow.

Resort spa – *re-sor-t sp-ar* – a **spa** establishment offering **treatments** at a vacation destination that also has other

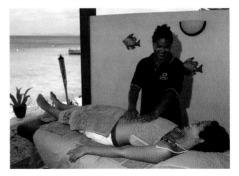

An example of a resort spa

facilities such as water sports, golf, tennis and children's activities.

Resources – re-sor-ses – the total of all the means available to a business to increase profit, e.g. equipment, products, time, assets and people.

Respiration – res-pi-ray-shon – the process of breathing in and out, which allows the *gaseous exchange* in the body, taking in *oxygen* and releasing *carbon dioxide*.

Respiratory system – res-pir-at-or-ee sis-t-em – the air passages, lungs and muscles that work together to move air in and out of the body. The respiratory system helps to oxygenate (add *oxygen* to) the blood and remove *carbon dioxide* and *metabolic waste* from the circulation. *Respiration* is achieved through the mouth, nose, *trachea*, *bronchi*, *bronchioles*, lungs, *alveoli* and *diaphragm*.

Retail – r-ee-tay-l – to sell goods in small quantities directly to the consumer or client.

Retailer – ree-tay-ler – a person or business that sells goods directly to the consumer or client.

Retinoic acid – ret-in-oh-ik as-id – a substance derived from vitamin A and incorporated into skin care products. It is used to treat *acne* and lessen the appearance of fine lines and *wrinkles*, *hyperpigmentation* and roughness of facial skin. The side effects are extreme sensitivity to sunlight, increased reddening of the skin and peeling.

Review – re-v-you – a critical article, survey or report or an inspection or examination. *Also to* look at something for a second time, to look back on something, to repeat or summarise.

Rheostat – ree-oh-st-at – an instrument that regulates *electric current*.

Rhinestones – r-eye-n-st-oh-n-s – tiny, metallic, flat-backed, multi-coloured crystals, used for nail art design. They are cut on the upper surface like a gem stone, with many sides, to add sparkle to the nails.

Rhomboid major – *rom-boy-d may-jor* – a diamond-shaped *muscle* beneath the **trapezius** in the upper back, attaching the *scapula* to the spinal **vertebrae**. It is the larger of the two rhomboid muscles and it retracts (pulls towards the **midline**) and rotates the scapula.

Rhomboid minor – *rom-boy-d m-eye-nor* – a **muscle** that is situated above and very close to the larger *rhomboid major* muscle and having the same actions.

Ribs – *ri-b-s* – the long curved bones that form the cage of bones surrounding the thorax (chest). They protect the lungs, heart and other internal organs in the thoracic (chest) cavity. (See the diagram on page 195.)

Ringworm – *rin-g-wer-m* – a highly contagious (spread by contact) fungal infection of the body. The *fungus* produces *enzymes* that break down the *keratin* in the skin causing characteristic circular, scaly, itching patches. The ring shape spreads outwards and the centre gradually heals, returning to normal skin colour. Ringworm is usually caused by a group of fungi called dermatophytes. Spores (reproductive structures) from the fungus may be picked up from another person, the soil, the environment, an animal or household objects. The Latin name of the ringworm fungus is *Tinea* and this is followed by the Latin term to describe the part of the body affected by the fungus, e.g. *Tinea corporis* (body), *Tinea capitis* (scalp), *Tinea unguium* (nail – see **onychomycosis**) and *Tinea pedis* (feet – see **athlete's foot**).

Risk – *ri-s-k* – danger of suffering harm.

Risorius – *ri-sor-ee-as* – a facial *muscle* – the **origin** is in the *masseter* muscle and the *insertion* is in the **orbicularis oris** muscle surrounding the mouth. It pulls the corners of the mouth outwards. (See the diagram on page 192.)

Roman bath – *r-oh-man ba-th* – an ancient building used for bathing with a series of hot, warm and cold pools. Roman baths still exist in their original form in some of the *spa* towns in the UK. Many of the new spas have adapted the principles and updated them to fit in with the latest trends.

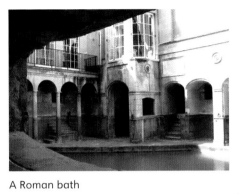

A Roman bath

Rosacea – *r-oh-say-sha* – a skin *disease* affecting the middle of the face. It causes persistent redness over the cheeks and nose, dilated (enlarged) *capillaries* that form fine red lines (telangiectasias) in the skin, and small spots. It occurs most commonly in adults aged between 30 and 50 and is made worse by *stress*, extremes of temperature and sun exposure. It affects more men than women. The *Heliobacter pylori* **bacteria** present in the **follicles** are thought to contribute to the development of rosacea. In extreme cases rhinophyma (enlarged nose and puffy cheeks) may occur.

Rosacea keratitis – *r-oh-say-sha ker-at-eye-t-is* – a complication of *rosacea* that affects the eyes. It begins with a burning and gritty sensation and if left untreated will damage the cornea (the transparent front surface of the eye) and impair vision.

Rosewater – *r-oh-s-w-or-ter* – a facial **toning lotion** obtained by steam distilling (extracting a substance from) the petals of roses.

Rotator cuff muscles – *r-oh-tay-tor-kuf mu-sel-s* – a group of four *muscles* situated around the shoulder joint and consisting of the subscapularis, teres minor, infraspinatus and supraspinatus. Their function is to keep the shoulder joint stable during movements of the arm. (See the diagram on page 202.)

Rules – *r-ool-s* – principles or regulations provided to guide an individual when carrying out procedures and in their behaviour and actions.

Salary – *sal-a-ree* – a fixed amount of money paid to an employee on a regular basis in return for work done.

Sales – *say-l-s* – revenue gained from selling goods and services.

Saline solution – *say-l-eye-n sol-oo-sh-on* – a liquid mixture of water and salt, usually one pint of water to one teaspoon of salt. It is used in electrical facial and body treatments to help conduct (carry) the *electric current*. When using a *galvanic unit*, the viscose sponges are soaked in saline solution, and when using a *faradic unit* for body treatment, the *electrodes* are dampened with saline solution before placing them on the skin.

Salon services – *sa-lon ser-vis-es* – a range of professional treatments and activities available in a beauty salon or spa.

Salt rub – *s-ol-t rub* – a wax, oil or cream containing sea salt used in *exfoliation*, leaving the skin feeling softer and smoother. Sometimes used together with *essential oils*.

Salycilic acid – *sal-i-sil-ik as-id* – a *beta hydroxy acid* that is an effective *exfoliant* but a mild irritant. It is prescribed by dermatologists (doctors specialising in skin complaints) for removing skin blemishes, and it also improves skin thickness, barrier functions and *collagen* production. It is used in small concentrations in skin care products to exfoliate the skin and penetrate deeper into the *follicles*, helping to remove *comedones* and *milia*.

Sanitise – *san-it-eye-s* – to make clean and hygienic (see *hygiene*).

Saponification – *sap-on-if-ik-ay-shon* – the breaking down of a fat by an alkali (see *alkaline*) to form soap. This occurs when the negative pole in *desincrustation* is applied to the skin. The alkaline reaction breaks down (*emulsifies*) the *sebum*, making it easier to remove.

Sartorius – *s-ar-tor-ee-us* – the longest *muscle* in the body. It runs down the length of the thigh from the hip to the *medial* side of the knee. (See the diagram on page 202.)

Saturator – *sat-you-ray-tor* – an *electrode* used in treatments using an indirect *high-frequency current*. It is held by the client to complete the electrical circuit.

Sauna – *s-or-na* – a small room or building with wooden seating, heated to a temperature of 80–100°C. Used originally for bathing and now also for physical and mental relaxation. Saunas have been used in Finland for at least 1,000 years and other cultures have similar sweat baths: the Turkish *hammam*, the Russian *bania* and the Native American sweat lodge or *inipi*.

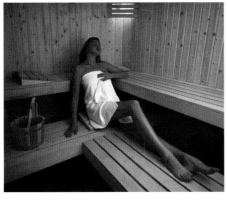

A sauna

Scab – *sk-ab* – a crust that forms over a wound as protection during the healing process. It is a coagulation (transformation of a liquid into a semi-solid form) of body fluids, which then hardens and becomes solid.

Scabies – *sk-ay-bee-s* – an infestation (attack by *parasites*) of the skin caused by a tiny itch mite (*Sarcoptes scabiei*) burrowing under the skin, especially around the hands and feet. It is characterised by intense itching, as a result of an *allergic* reaction to the mite, and a *rash* caused by the mite tunnelling under the skin and leaving tracks. As the mite burrows it lays eggs and several days later these hatch and the young mites begin to move. It is a highly contagious (spread by contact) condition requiring medical treatment.

Scale – *sk-ay-l* – an accumulation of epidermal flakes (dead skin cells), which may be dry or greasy. Scale indicates an abnormal process of *keratinisation*.

Scaphoid – *ska-foy-d* – a small bone in the wrist. (See the diagram on page 197.)

Scapula – *sk-ap-you-la* (plural **scapulae** – *sk-ap-you-lie*) – the shoulder blade. A flat, triangular bone that forms the back *(continued)* part of the **shoulder girdle**. There are two scapulae, one at each side of the spine. (See the diagram on page 195.)

Scar – *sk-ar* – a mark left on the skin. They are areas of fibrous tissue (**connective tissue** with a high concentration of **collagen** fibres) that have replaced healthy skin after destruction of **cells** in the **epidermis** through injury or disease. Scarring is a natural part of the healing process when the skin lays down new collagen fibres to mend the damaged tissue. This new skin has a different texture and quality from the surrounding tissue.

Schedule – *sh-ed-you-l* – a timetable, plan or list of activities to be carried out in a given time to achieve an objective. A schedule provides a logical sequence of activities and the time required to complete each activity.

Scoliosis – *sk-oh-lee-oh-sis* – an abnormal **lateral** (sideways) curvature (curving) of the spine.

Sculptured nails – *sk-ul-p-t-your-d n-ay-ls* – see **acrylic nails**.

Seasonal promotions – *see-s-on-al pr-o-m-oh-shon-s* – special offers that change according to the time of year, e.g. Mother's Day, post-Christmas or pre-summer packages.

Sebaceous glands – *seb-ay-shus gl-and-s* – **exocrine glands** found in the **dermis** all over the body apart from the soles of the feet and palms of the hands. They secrete **sebum** and are situated next to **hair follicles**. The sebaceous gland, the hair and the follicle together are called the **pilosebaceous unit**. Sebaceous glands are classed as **holocrine glands**, as sebum is produced within specialised cells and secreted when the cells lining the sebaceous gland break down. **Sebum** provides a waterproof coating on the hair and skin and helps to reduce the growth of micro-organisms (organisms too small to be seen by the naked eye) on the skin. (See the diagram on page 189.)

Seborrhoea – *seb-or-ee-a* – excessively **oily skin** caused by overactive **sebaceous glands** producing large amounts of **sebum**, which makes the skin look shiny. In some cases it may result in **acne**.

Sebum – *see-bum* – an oily *secretion* produced by the *sebaceous glands* to waterproof the skin and hair and protect the skin from *infection* by *bacteria* and *fungi*. It is made up of lipids (fat) and the debris of dead, fat-producing cells. Excess sebum is associated with *oily skin* and *acne*. This is particularly common in adolescents due to the increased levels of sex *hormones* (*androgens*) which stimulate sebum production. Lack of sebum is common in middle and older age and leads to skin dryness and *wrinkle* formation.

Secretion – *se-kree-sh-on* – the substance produced and released by a *gland*. *Also* the act of releasing a substance.

Security – *se-k-yor-it-ee* – freedom from danger. *Also* precautions taken to make something safe. *Also* a department in an organisation that is responsible for protection or safety.

Self-tan – *se-l-f tan* – a liquid, cream, spray or *gel* formulation for home use to colour the skin.

Self-tanning – *se-l-f tan-in-g* – application of a false tan product to oneself.

Senior therapist – *see-nee-or th-er-ap-ist* – an experienced therapist with a higher position in the organisation.

Sensitiser – *sen-sit-eyes-er* – a substance that makes the skin more sensitive, so that the next exposure to that substance will cause an *allergic* reaction.

Sensitive skin – *sen-sit-iv sk-in* – a skin condition that reacts quickly to external stimuli such as heat and cold. It is characterised by its pale, translucent (semi-transparent) colour, dry *epidermis* and fine texture. It is prone to *allergic* reaction, sometimes becoming red and blotchy, and is easily irritated by certain products and perfumes.

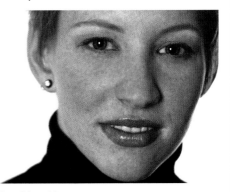

Sensitive skin

153

Sensory nerves – *sen-s-or-ee ner-v-s* – **cells** that form part of the **nervous system** and that receive and pass on information to do with the senses, such as pain, heat, pressure and movement. They are **afferent** as they carry nerve impulses from sense organs towards the **central nervous system**.

Sepsis – *sep-sis* – the presence of pus-forming **bacteria** or their **toxins** in the blood or **tissues**.

Septic – *sep-tik* – infected with germs.

Septum – *se-p-tum* – a dividing wall, partition or **membrane** that separates two cavities (spaces), e.g. the nasal septum dividing the nose into two nostrils or the septum of the heart dividing the right and left **ventricles**.

Services – *ser-vis-is* – professional activities and processes that are offered to others to provide **benefits**, e.g. a **manicure**, **pedicure**, **aromatherapy** massage or **electrical facial**.

Setting – *set-tin-g* – tightening or hardening of a substance, e.g. a clay **face mask** is a setting mask.

Shader – *sh-ay-d-er* – a **cosmetic** product used to obscure or darken an area, or to provide contour and shape to the face.

Sharps box – *sh-ar-p-s bo-ks* – a yellow, rigid container used especially for the safe disposal of any sharp objects such as broken glass, needles and pipettes. The boxes come in a range of sizes, including small portable containers, and have a **hazard** symbol displayed clearly, with a brief written description of their use.

Shaving – *sh-ay-v-in-g* – a method of removing superfluous hair with a razor.

Shirodhara – *sh-i-rod-ar-a* – an Ayurvedic (see **Ayurveda**) facial treatment during which a stream of oil is poured on the forehead (an area referred to as 'the third eye') to aid relaxation of mind and body.

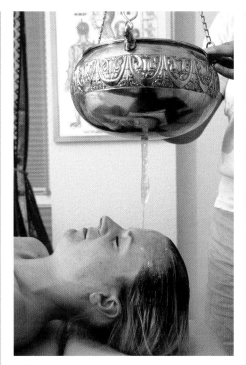
Shirodhara treatment

Shoulder girdle – *show-l-der g-er-dul* – the bones that connect the arms to the breastbone (*sternum*), consisting of the *clavicle* and the *scapulae*.

Shower – *sh-ow-er* – a form of *hydrotherapy*. Water is sprayed over the body from an overhead perforated nozzle. It may be used to cleanse or warm the body before a *treatment*, to remove products from the skin during treatment, to cool down the body during treatment or to remove

sweat and waste products after treatment. The shower can be adapted to provide other hydrotherapy treatments such as the *vichy shower* or power jet massage.

Silk wrap – *si-lk rap* – a thin layer used in the application of false nails or to strengthen a natural nail. It is made from silk, a tightly woven natural material, which is strong and light in weight. It becomes transparent when adhesive is applied, providing a smooth finish. Also known as a silk overlay.

Simulation – *sim-you-lay-shon* – the imitation or acting out of a certain process or scenario for training purposes.

Skeletal muscle – *sk-e-lee-t-al mus-sel* – a type of striated (striped), voluntary (under conscious control by the brain) muscle attached to the skeleton. It is the most common of the three types of muscle in the human body. Skeletal muscles are contractile (capable of *contraction*). They produce movement by applying force to bones and *joints*, maintain *posture* and generate *(continued)*

155

heat. They have one end (the origin) attached to a relatively stationary bone and the other end (the insertion) attached across a joint to the bone that moves. Also known as **voluntary muscle** and **striated muscle**.

Skeletal system – *sk-e-lee-t-al sis-t-m* – a rigid framework, made up of 206 bones, that shapes and supports the body. Vital organs are protected by the skeletal system and movement is achieved by interaction with the **muscular system**. Blood **cells** are produced in the bone marrow (soft tissue in the centre of bones) and bones act as a reservoir (store) for minerals such as calcium and phosphorous. The skeleton is divided into the **axial skeleton**, consisting of the **skull**, **sternum**, **ribs** and spinal column (see **vertebra**), and the **appendicular skeleton**, consisting of the bones of the arm and hand, leg and foot, **pelvic girdle** and **shoulder girdle**. (See the diagram on page 195.)

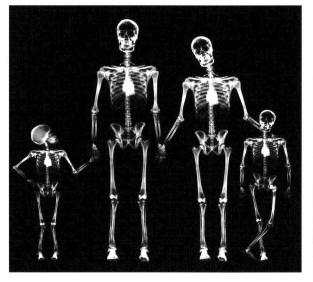

The skeletal system

Skin – *sk-in* – the largest organ in the body. It provides the external covering of the body, also known as the **integumentary system** (consisting of skin, hair, nails and **glands**). It has three layers: the **epidermis**, **dermis** and **subcutaneous layer**. It protects underlying organs and **muscles**. Other functions are insulation (preventing heat loss), temperature regulation, protection against pathogens (disease-producing organisms), sensation (feeling), **vitamin** production, **absorption**, **secretion** and **excretion**. (See the diagram on page 189.)

Skin analysis – *sk-in an-al-i-sis* – a careful examination of the skin by the therapist to identify the requirements of the client for treatment and home care. This procedure is carried out before any facial treatment and the therapist will assess the colour, texture, pore size, *sebaceous gland* activity, skin condition, *elasticity*, blemishes and muscle tone.

Skin care routine – *sk-in ker roo-tee-n* – regular use of products and techniques in order to maintain or improve *skin condition*.

Skin colour – *sk-in ku-ler* – there are many different colours of skin, varying in tone from almost colourless, with a pink hue from the blood in the skin, to very dark. Colour is determined by the amount and type of *melanin* present in the skin. Generally speaking, people with ancestors from sunnier regions have darker skin than those from areas that have less or very little sunlight.

Skin condition – *sk-in kon-di-sh-on* – the appearance, texture and state of health of the skin at a given time.

Skin freshener – *sk-in fr-esh-en-er* – the mildest form of *astringent* used to tone the skin, made from soothing ingredients such as *rosewater*.

Skin functions – *sk-in fun-k-shon-s* – the physiological activities (the normal processes) of the skin. These include protection, heat regulation, sensation (feeling), *secretion*, *excretion*, *absorption* and *vitamin* production.

Skin resurfacing – *sk-in ree-ser-fus-ing* – treatments used to change the surface texture of the skin, including *chemical peels*, *microdermabrasion* and *laser* resurfacing.

Skin rolling – *sk-in r-oh-lin-g* – a pressure *massage* manipulation in which the *tissue* is lifted and rolled against underlying bone. Working transversely (across the body), the tissues are grasped firmly between fingers and thumbs and the thumbs are used to roll the skin and muscle away. This movement stimulates blood and skin, releases tension and relaxes the client.

Skin sensitivity test – *sk-in sen-sit-iv-it-ee t-es-t* – an assessment of the ability of the skin to react to a stimulus. This may be performed in two ways: by tactile (involving touch) methods using a soft and sharp object, or thermally (involving heat) using hot and cold test tubes.

Skin tag – *sk-in tag* – a common *benign* condition. It is a loose growth of skin projecting from the surrounding surface. It may be smooth or irregular in shape, flesh-coloured or pigmented (coloured). Tags occur most often on the eyelids, neck, armpits and upper chest area. Also known as a cutaneous papilloma.

Skin tonic – *sk-in ton-ik* – a form of *astringent* used to remove surface grease, tighten the *pores* and stimulate the skin.

Skin type – *sk-in t-eye-p* – a classification of the skin gained during *skin analysis*, to help determine the products to use and treatments to provide. Each type has different characteristics. The four main types are *dry*, *oily*, *combination* and *normal*. *Sensitive*, *dehydrated* and *mature* are also classifications of skin type or *skin condition*.

Skin warming – *sk-in w-or-min-g* – methods of gently heating the skin using hot towels, *infrared* or a facial steamer to prepare the skin for further treatment.

Skull – *sk-u-l* – the bony framework of the head that encloses and protects the brain and supports the face. It is made up of the cranium and facial bones. The cranium bones: 1 frontal, 2 parietal, 2 temporal, 1 occipital, 1 ethmoid, 1 sphenoid. The facial bones: 2 lacrimal, 4 nasal, 1 vomer, 1 maxilla, 1 mandible, 2 zygomatic and 2 palatine. (See the diagram on page 196.)

Smooth muscle – *sm-oo-th mus-sel* – a type of *involuntary muscle* found in the walls of hollow organs such as *blood vessels*, the digestive tract (the mouth, *oesophagus*, stomach and intestines), the bladder and *uterus*.

Soapless cleanser – *s-oh-p-less klen-s-er* – a product with a combination of water and oils that is used to remove dirt and debris from the skin without stripping it of moisture.

Sole trader – *s-oh-l tr-ay-der* – the legal business status when one person sets up a business on their own. It is the simplest way to run a business, as the sole trader makes all the decisions and keeps all the profit. However, the sole trader is personally liable for all debts.

Soleus – *s-oh-lee-us* – a powerful *muscle* in the *posterior* lower leg, running from the knee to the heel. It is vital in standing, running, walking and dancing. Its action is *plantarflexion* of the foot. (See the diagram on page 202.)

Solvent – *sol-v-en-t* – a substance that dissolves another substance to form a solution (e.g. *acetone* in nail polish remover).

Solvent extraction – *sol-v-en-t x-trak-sh-on* – a method of obtaining *essential oils* from plants. The raw materials are covered with a *solvent* and heated to extract the essential oil. The liquid is then filtered, leaving a paste of fragranced wax that is mixed with alcohol and distilled at low temperatures. The alcohol absorbs the fragrance and when the alcohol is evaporated off the aromatic essential oil remains.

Somatic nervous system – *so-mat-ik ner-v-us sis-t-em* – the part of the *peripheral nervous system* involved in the voluntary control of body movement through the action of *skeletal muscles*. It is also involved in receiving external (from outside the body) stimuli (things that cause a response) through the five senses. It consists of *afferent* fibres that receive information and *efferent* fibres that transmit information and are responsible for muscle *contraction*. (See the diagram on page 201.)

Somatotrophin – *so-mat-o-trof-in* – a growth *hormone* secreted (released) by the *anterior* lobe (section) of the *pituitary gland*. It causes *cells* to grow and multiply. Also known as growth hormone (GH).

Spa – *sp-ar* – a place of naturally occurring mineral waters. The name of a town in Belgium that attracted people for the benefits derived from its healing water. Today it is *(continued)* the term used to describe a luxurious resort offering beauty and holistic therapies.

Spatula – *sp-at-you-la* – a small, flat, wooden or plastic implement for removing creams and other products from containers to prevent *cross-infection*.

Special offer – *sp-esh-al of-er* – to make available something that is exceptional or different from the ordinary for a specific purpose, e.g. to increase turnover, attract new clients to a business or sell off products reaching their sell-by date. Offers may include a special *discount*, 'buy one get one free', a course of treatments at a reduced rate, or earning points on all products and treatments purchased to be exchanged for goods or treatments.

Special senses – *sp-e-sh-l sen-ses* – specialised functions located in particular organs of the body, which make it possible to experience the environment, including sight (eyes), hearing (ears), smell (nose), taste (tongue) and touch (skin).

Sphincter – *sf-ink-t-er* – a circular *muscle* that constricts (narrows) a body passage, e.g. the *orbicularis oris* muscle around the mouth and the pyloric sphincter at the lower end of the stomach, which allows food to pass from the stomach to the *duodenum*.

Spider naevus – *sp-eye-der nee-vus* – a small *benign tumour* consisting mainly of dilated (enlarged) or newly formed blood vessels (telangiectases). The name comes from the appearance of the central vessel resembling the body of a spider with fine radiating vessels resembling the legs.

Splenius capitis – *sp-len-ee-us cap-it-is* – the deep *muscle* located at the base of the back of the neck, from behind the ear to the thoracic (in the chest) *vertebrae*. It *extends*, rotates and laterally (sideways) *flexes* the head.

Splenius cervicus – *sp-len-ee-us ser-vik-us* – the *muscle* at the back of the neck from the top of the cervical (in the neck) *vertebrae* to the thoracic (in the chest) vertebrae. It *extends* and rotates the cervical spine.

Squamous cell carcinoma – *sk-w-ay-mus sel kar-sin-oh-ma* – a cancerous *tumour* which affects the *epidermis*. It is initially painless but may develop ulcers (open sores) that do not heal and then become painful. It often forms from an area of sun-damaged skin on the face, neck or hands.

Staff meeting – *st-af mee-tin-g* – a gathering of the employees of a business to discuss relevant issues or for some other common purpose.

Staphylococcus – *st-af-il-oh-cok-us* – a common type of *bacterium* that lives on the skin and *membranes* of the body. It is capable of causing *infection* through *toxin* production or invasion of the skin in conditions such as *impetigo* and *folliculitis*, and secondary infection of wounds caused by *scabies* and *eczema*.

Statutory – *stat-you-tor-ee* – authorised by statute (law). Disobeying statutory laws may be legally punishable.

Steam bath – *st-ee-m ba-th* – varying from a small cabinet to a large room that is filled with steam, and is used to relax the body, soften and cleanse the skin. Popular in *spas* and salons, it is an excellent preparatory treatment before other body treatments. Specialised steam baths include *hammams*, *rasul* and *serail* rooms, which are tiled rooms in which the bather sits after coating themselves in a special mud and then showers to remove the mud. Aroma grottos are a type of steam bath in which *essential oils* are added to the steam for their beneficial effects, e.g. lavender to soothe or eucalyptus to help breathe more easily.

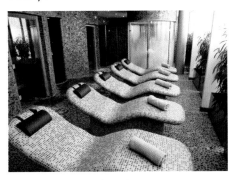

Steam room and relaxation area

Steam distillation – *st-ee-m dis-til-ay-shon* – a method used in the manufacture and extraction

161

of *essential oils*. Steam is forced over the flowers or plants, releasing aromatic *molecules*. This steam, containing the *fragrance*, is then passed through a cooling system, condensing it into a liquid, which is separated into the essential oil and water.

Sterilisation – *st-e-ril-eye-say-shon* – the complete destruction of *bacteria*, *viruses* and *fungi*. The *autoclave* is the most effective method of sterilisation. Other methods are *irradiation* and chemical disinfectants.

Sterilise – *st-e-ril-eye-s* – to completely destroy *bacteria*, *viruses* and *fungi*.

Sternocleidomastoid – *st-er-no-kl-eye-doh-mas-toy-d* – a thick *muscle* running from the *sternum* and *clavicle* to the occipital bone (bone at the base of the *skull*) on either side of the neck. *Contraction* of one side alone turns the head; both sides contracting together *flexes* the neck and bends the head. (See the diagram on page 192.)

Sternum – *st-er-num* – the breastbone. A long, flat bone located in the centre of the thorax (chest). Together with the *ribs* it helps to protect the heart and lungs. (See the diagram on page 195.)

Steroid – *st-e-roy-d* – a type of *hormone* produced by the adrenal *cortex* (see *adrenal gland*) and by the *ovaries* and *testes*.

Stock control – *st-ok kon-tr-oh-l* – procedures used to ensure that the right amount of supplies are available in the right place at the right time to meet the needs of the business and the clients. It also ensures that capital (the money of a business) is not tied up unnecessarily.

Stock taking – *st-ok tay-kin-g* – a procedure used to maintain adequate levels of supplies. An appointed person counts the numbers of each item available for use. Depending on the information gathered, an order can be placed for items that are no longer available or are available only in small numbers.

Stratum corneum – *st-r-ar-tum kor-nee-um* – the top layer of the *epidermis*, made up of dead, flat skin *cells* with no *nucleus* that are constantly being shed from the surface of the skin. These cells contain the protein **keratin** that helps prevent water evaporation and also absorbs water. (See the diagram on page 189.) Also known as the horny layer.

Stratum germinativum – *st-r-ar-tum jer-min-ay-tiv-um* – the deepest layer of the **epidermis**, consisting of a single layer of **keratinocytes** (specialised cells that produce **keratin**). It lies immediately above the **dermis**, from which it receives nutrient fluid from the **blood vessels**. It is in this layer that the cells undergo rapid cell division (**mitosis**). Approximately 25 per cent of cells in this layer are **melanocytes** which produce **melanin**, providing colour for skin and hair. (See the diagram on page 189.) Also known as the basal layer or germinative layer.

Stratum granulosum – *st-r-ar-tum gran-you-lo-sum* – a layer of the **epidermis**, lying between the **stratum spinosum** and the **stratum lucidum**. The final stages of **keratinisation** take place in this layer. The cells flatten as the **nucleus** begins to disintegrate and there is a loss of fluids which contributes to the transformation of cells into **keratin**. The keratin

helps form a waterproof barrier that prevents fluid loss from the body. (See the diagram on page 189.) Also known as the granular layer.

Stratum lucidum – *st-r-ar-tum loo-sid-um* – a layer of the **epidermis** situated between the **stratum corneum** and the **stratum granulosum**. It is a thin layer of clear, flat, dead skin cells. It is more evident on the thickest areas of skin – the palms of the hands and the soles of the feet. This layer is often referred to as the 'barrier' layer as it contains an oily substance that controls the transmission of water. (See the diagram on page 189.) Also known as the transparent layer.

Stratum spinosum – *st-r-ar-tum spin-oh sum* – a layer of the **epidermis** just above the **stratum germinativum**. The **keratinocytes** in this layer have 'spiky' projections called desmosomes which attach cells to each other. The **keratinisation** process begins in this layer, changing living cells with a **nucleus** into a hard, durable **protein** called **keratin**. This layer also contains **Langerhans' cells**, which attach themselves to foreign bodies (objects coming from *(continued)*

163

outside the body) that enter the skin and alert the *immune system* to their presence. (See the diagram on page 189.) Also known as the prickle cell layer.

Strawberry mark – *st-r-or-be-ree m-ar-k* – a soft, raised swelling on the skin, bright red in colour and sometimes resembling a strawberry. It appears in the first month after birth. The cause is not fully understood but the mark is a *benign* overgrowth of blood vessels in the skin that shrinks slowly with age, disappearing altogether in many cases. Also known as strawberry *naevus* or infantile haemangioma.

Strength – *st-r-en-g-th* – an asset or good quality or attribute.

Streptococci – *st-rep-t-kok-ee* – *bacteria* that cause a number of *infections*, including 'Strep throat', *impetigo* and scarlet fever.

Stress – *st-res* – a state of excessive tension that is harmful to the body.

Stress management – *st-res man-aj-men-t* – taking measures to reduce *stress* and combat its

negative effects, using a combination of physical exercise, deep relaxation, visualisation techniques and therapeutic treatments.

Stretch marks – *st-r-et-ch m-ar-k-s* – small marks or lines on the skin that look like thin, stretched *tissue*. They appear when a person puts on or loses weight rapidly, or after pregnancy. They are more common on areas of fat storage, such as the *abdomen*, breasts, upper arms, thighs and buttocks. On a pale skin they begin as slightly raised red marks that turn purple before slowly fading to a silvery colour. They occur in the *dermis* where *collagen* and **elastin** fibres become thinner and less elastic (see *elasticity*). When the fibres break the skin appears thinner and these areas show as stretch marks. Also known as striae.

Striated muscle – *st-r-eye-ay-ted mus-el* – see *skeletal muscle*.

Stye – *st-eye* – an *inflammation* of the *sebaceous glands* at the base of the eyelashes, caused by a bacterial *infection*. It looks tender and red and has a pus-filled centre. Also known as *hordeolum*.

Subcutaneous layer – *sub-q-tay-nee-us lay-er* – the deepest layer of the skin, lying below the *dermis*. It is made up of loose *connective tissue*, *adipose tissue*, *blood vessels* and *nerves*. Its functions include insulation (preventing heat loss), protection and storage of *nutrients*. (See the diagram on page 189.)

Sudoriferous glands – *soo-d-or-if-er-us gl-and-s* – see *sweat glands*.

Sugaring – *sh-ug-ar-in-g* – a technique used to remove superfluous hair that has been popular in the Middle East for centuries. Originally, sugar, water and lemon juice were boiled and then cooled to form a workable paste. Today, similar products have been developed that are safer to use. The paste is rolled into a ball, flattened onto the skin and then quickly stripped away, removing the hair at the root. It is thought to be gentler on the skin than *wax*, as it is water-soluble (dissolves in water) and the natural ingredients do not irritate a *sensitive skin*.

Sun protection factor (SPF) – *sun pr-oh-tek-shon fak-t-or* – a number given to a *sunscreen* product that identifies its ability to protect the skin from sunburn. The number represents how many times longer a person can stay in the sun without burning if the product is applied. It is a measure of protection against *ultraviolet radiation* (UVB rays are the rays responsible for causing sunburn).

Sunburn – *sun b-er-n* – a burn to the skin caused by over-exposure to *ultraviolet radiation* from the sun's rays or other sources, such as equipment used in tanning salons. In the *stratum germinativum* of the *epidermis* the *Langerhans' cells* (which play an important part in the *immune system*) are reduced in number. Mild symptoms are *erythema*, tender skin, being hot to the touch, feeling unwell and dizziness. In more serious cases blistering occurs, accompanied by pain and then skin peeling. The long-term consequences to the skin are premature ageing and *wrinkles*, *pigmented* areas of skin, *lesions* such as actinic keratoses and the development of skin cancer.

Sunscreen – *sun sk-ree-n* – a substance applied to the skin that is formulated to prevent sunburn and reduce skin damage by absorbing or reflecting harmful *ultraviolet radiation*. A broad spectrum sunscreen is advised to protect from both UVA and UVB rays. The protection from UVB is indicated by a number between 1 and 30+. Protection from UVA rays is indicated with a star rating. Sunscreens come in several different formulations: oil, cream, *gel*, wipes or spray.

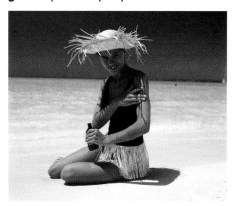

Applying sunscreen

Superficial cleanse – *soo-per-fi-sh-l klen-s* – cleansing the skin at the beginning of a *facial* after removing eye and lip *makeup*. This is always carried out, even on a client who is not wearing makeup, and is followed by a deep cleanse using deeper relaxing movements.

Superfluous – *soo-per-floo-us* – excessive, more than is required, unwanted.

Superior – *soo-pee-ree-or* – situated above, higher in station or rank, of a higher grade or quality or above average in excellence.

Supervisor – *soo-per-v-eyes-or* – a person who organises, monitors and controls the work done by others.

Supination – *soo-pin-ay-shon* – rotation of the forearm so that the palm faces forward or up.

Supine – *soo-p-eye-n* – lying face upwards.

Supplier – *su-pl-eye-er* – a person or company that provides goods.

Surgical spirit – *ser-jik-al sp-i-rit* – a colourless mixture of ethanol and methanol (cleaning chemicals) used to clean and *sterilise* surfaces.

Sweat – *sw-et* – a salty, watery solution produced by *sweat glands* and secreted (released) through numerous microscopic channels that open onto the surface of the skin. This helps to control body temperature as the sweat evaporates (disappears) from the surface of the skin and cools the body down. It also aids in the removal of waste products from the body. As *sebum* from the *sebaceous glands* and sweat mix on the skin surface, they form a protective layer called the *acid mantle*.

Sweat glands – *sw-et gl-and-s* – glands in the *dermis* that excrete (remove from the body) waste products through *sweat* and help to control body temperature. They are classified as *apocrine* and *eccrine glands*. Also known as *sudoriferous glands*.

Swedish massage – *s-wee-di-sh mass-ar-j* – a classical European *massage* using techniques developed by Pehr Henrik Ling (1776–1839), a Swedish gymnastics coach. It is designed to relax *muscles* by applying pressure against deeper muscles and bones. Swedish massage helps the recovery of strained muscles by flushing *lactic acid* (produced in muscles during exercise), uric acid (a product of protein *metabolism*) and *metabolic waste* out of the *tissues*. The massage techniques used are *effleurage*, *petrissage*, *vibrations*, *frictions* and *percussion*. These French names were given to the movements by Johann Georg Mezger (1838–1909), a Dutch physician. The main *benefits* are an increase in circulation, keeping *ligaments* and *tendons* supple, reducing emotional and physical *stress*, soothing or stimulating the nerves and promoting health and well-being.

SWOT analysis – *sw-ot an-al-i-sis* – an examination of the internal strengths and weaknesses and the external opportunities and threats facing a business.

Sympathetic nervous system – *sim-path-e-tik ner-vus sis-t-em* – part of the *autonomic nervous system* that is activated under conditions of *stress* and speeds up the heartbeat, contracts (narrows) the *blood vessels*, regulates the function of the sweat *glands* and stimulates the *secretion* of *glucose* in the liver.

Synapse – *s-eye-naps* – the area between **neurons** where **nerve** impulses (signals) are transmitted and received.

Synergy – *sin-er-jee* – the interaction of two or more agents so that their combined effect is greater than the sum of their individual effects.

Synovial joint – *s-eye-no-vee-al joy-n-t* – the most common type of joint in the body. A moveable **joint** that contains a lubricating (slippery) liquid called synovial fluid, which reduces friction of the bones during movement. There are several types of synovial joint: ball and socket joints (e.g. hip and shoulder); gliding joints, which occur between the surfaces of two flat bones held together by **ligaments** (e.g. wrist and ankle); hinge joints (e.g. knee and elbow); ellipsoid joints, which are similar to ball and socket joints and allow the same kind of movement but to a lesser degree (e.g. at the end of the index finger); pivot joints, which allow rotation in the socket (e.g. the atlas and axis in the neck allow the head to turn); and saddle joints, which have limited rotation (e.g. in the thumb).

Synthesis – *sin-th-e-sis* – the combining of separate elements or substances to form a whole.

Systemic circulation – *sis-tem-ik ser-q-lay-shon* – the part of the **circulatory system** that carries **oxygenated blood** away from the **heart** to the body and returns **deoxygenated blood** back to the heart. (See the diagram on page 199.)

Systemic medical condition – *sis-tem-ik med-ik-al kon-di-shon* – a disease or disorder of a body system that affects the entire body.

Systolic pressure – *sis-t-o-lik pre-sh-er* – the **blood pressure** when the heart is contracting (thickening and tightening in order to pump the blood), the first number recorded in a blood pressure reading.

Tactile skin sensitivity test –
*tak-t-eye-l sk-in sen-sit-iv-it-ee
tes-t* – a safety precaution used
before electrical treatments to
check the amount of feeling in the
client's skin. A piece of cotton
wool and the end of an orange
stick are applied alternately to the
skin to make sure that the client
can feel the difference between
the two.

Talc – *ta-l-k* – a naturally
occurring fine mineral powder
used as a lubricant (a substance
that allows ease of movement) on
the skin for manual or gyratory
vibratory massage (see *gyratory
massager*).

Talus – *tal-us* – the second
largest *tarsal bone* in the foot,
connecting the leg to the foot. It
articulates (moves at a *joint*) with
the *tibia*, *fibula*, *calcaneus* and
navicular bones. (See the diagram
on page 197.)

Tapotement – *tap-oh-t-men-t* –
see *percussion*.

Target cell – *tar-get sel* – a *cell*
that responds to a *hormone*
because it contains receptors
(endings that are sensitive to a

messenger) for that particular
hormone.

Targets – *tar-get-s* – desired
goals, which may be set to
encourage increased production,
to provide motivation or to gain a
reward.

Tarsal bones – *tar-sal b-oh-n-s*
– seven bones in the foot: 1 *talus*,
1 *calcaneus* (heel), 3 *cuneiform*, 1
cuboid and 1 *navicular*. (See the
diagram on page 197.)

Tax – *t-ax* – a sum of money
paid to the government for
services. Tax is paid on income,
property, inheritance and
business. Tax is also paid through
VAT, excise duty, insurance
premium tax, petrol tax and
stamp duty when buying a house.

Team – *t-ee-m* – a group of
people working towards a
common goal for mutual benefit.

Technical skill – *tek-nik-al sk-il*
– a competence relevant to a
particular profession, which
requires special training and
experience.

Telangiectasia – *tel-an-jee-ek-
tay-sh-a* – a collection of* (continued)*

169

distended (increased in size) **blood vessels** in the skin, usually with a central spot and a spidery appearance.

Telogen – *tel-o-jen* – the resting phase in the development of a **hair follicle**. Telogen hairs have a clubbed or bulbous tip and last for several months before falling out.

Temperature gauge – *tem-pe-rat-y-or gay-j* – an implement used to assess or measure levels of heat.

Temporalis – *tem-p-or-ar-lis* – a facial muscle extending from the temple to the jawbone, the action of which is to raise the **mandible** and close the jaws. (See the diagram on page 192.)

Temporal bone – *tem-p-or-al b-oh-n* – a bone situated at the side and base of the skull, which encloses the organs of hearing and balance. (See the diagram on page 196.)

Tendon – *ten-don* – a band of fibrous (made up of fibres) **connective tissue** that connects muscle to bone.

Tendonitis – *ten-don-eye-t-is* – **inflammation** of a **tendon**.

Tepidarium – *tep-id-er-ee-um* – a warm room in the original Roman baths, used for relaxation and massage with oils, before further heat treatment. In modern **spas** this room is often the relaxation room used before, during and after the treatment.

Terminal hair – *t-er-min-al her* – a mature hair, which is generally longer, thicker and coarser than **vellus hair**.

Testes – *tes-tees* – the male **gonads**, part of the male reproductive system. They are **endocrine glands** that secrete (release) **androgens** (the most important of which is **testosterone**), which stimulate the development and maintenance of the male sexual characteristics: hair growth on the body, enlargement of the larynx (upper throat containing the vocal cords) and production of sperm. (See the diagram on page 200.) Also known as testicles.

Testosterone – *tes-tos-t-er-oh-n* – the principal male sex **hormone**.

Thai massage – *t-eye mas-ar-j* – a *therapy* performed on a client, who should be wearing loose-fitting clothing. It includes passive, yoga-like stretching movements and pressure-point massage along the body's major energy channels, to release blocked energy and tension while helping relaxation.

Thalassotherapy – *th-al-as-oh-th-er-a-pee* – a *treatment* that combines the use of sea water, mineral-rich mud and seaweed with *hydrotherapy*. It is offered in many *spas*, originally to improve health, digestive problems and muscular disorders, but more recently for modern ailments such as *stress*, fatigue, *joint* and back pain. It is believed that all natural elements exist in the sea and the chemical composition of sea water is similar to human *plasma*. The iodine (a mineral necessary for *metabolism*) content is a powerful natural *antiseptic* and seaweed is a potent detoxifier (an agent that helps eliminate *toxins*).

Therapeutic – *th-e-rap-you-tic* – having the power to heal or improve well-being.

Therapy – *th-e-rap-ee* – a procedure that has beneficial effects on the client and helps to remedy a problem, or a healing power or quality.

Thermal – *th-er-mal* – relating to heat or capable of creating or retaining heat.

Thermal mask – *th-er-mal m-as-k* – a specialised clay skin preparation. When mixed with warm water and applied to the skin, the mask heats further to soothe and soften the skin. A special cream is massaged into the skin before the mask is applied. As the mask hardens a chemical reaction occurs to create the heat and warm the skin, allowing deeper penetration of the cream.

Thermal mittens – *th-er-mal mit-ten-s* – heated mittens used in a luxury *manicure* to apply heat, allow quicker penetration (reaching a certain depth) of *moisturisers* and soothe aching *joints*.

Thermal skin test – *th-er-mal sk-in tes-t* – the use of hot and cold to test skin sensitivity to heat. Two test tubes are filled, *(continued)* one with cold water and the other with warm water. The test tubes are placed alternately on the client's skin and the client is asked to say which one is cold and which one is warm. This test should be used before applying heat to the client's skin.

Thermocoagulation – *th-er-mo-ko-ag-you-lay-shon* – coagulation (change from a fluid to a thickened semi-solid form) by means of *high-frequency currents*.

Thermolysis – *th-er-mol-i-sis* – the change of a complex chemical substance into its simpler parts by means of heat. Also destruction of *tissues* by means of heat.

Thermostat – *th-er-m-oh-st-at* – a device for maintaining a constant set temperature.

Thoracic duct – *th-or-ass-ik duk-t* – a major *lymph vessel*, starting in front of the lower lumbar (in the lower back) *vertebrae*. At the bottom end of the thoracic duct there is the cisterna chyli (an enlarged lymph vessel situated in the *abdomen* which receives and temporarily stores *lymph*). The thoracic duct carries lymph from the lower limbs, pelvis, abdomen and lower chest up to a large *vein* in the chest, where the lymph is returned to the bloodstream. (See the diagram on page 199.)

Threading – *th-red-in-g* – a method of temporarily removing *superfluous* hair using cotton thread, a skill originating in the Middle East and Asia.

Thymus gland – *th-eye-mus gl-and* – an *endocrine gland* located in the upper *anterior* chest behind the *sternum*. It plays an important role in the development of the *immune system*. *Lymphocytes*, which are produced in the bone marrow, migrate (travel) to the thymus gland where they mature, multiply and become T cells (which are essential in fighting infections). (See the diagram on page 200.)

Thyroid gland – *th-eye-roy-d gl-and* – an *endocrine gland* located in the middle of the lower neck below the voice box and just above the *clavicles* (collar bones). It regulates the body's *metabolic rate* and influences the growth of the body. It secretes (releases) *thyroxin* – if this is over-produced it causes *hyperthyroidism*. Graves' disease is the most commom cause of hyperthyroidism – symptoms include protrusion (bulging) of the eyeballs. Under-*secretion* causes cretinism (stunted mental and physical growth) in children or myxoedema in middle age (characterised by thick skin, mental problems, low *metabolism*, weight gain and hair loss). (See the diagram on page 200.)

Thyroxin – *th-eye-rox-in* – a *hormone* produced by the *thyroid gland* that acts on the body by increasing the *metabolic rate*.

Tibia – *tib-ee-a* – the inner of the two bones of the lower leg, extends from the knee to the ankle and joins with the *femur* and *talus*. (See the diagram on page 195.)

Tibialis anterior – *tib-ee-ay-lis ant-ee-ree-or* – *muscle* on the front of the lower leg, running down the outside of the shin, from just below the knee to the base of the first *metatarsal*. Its action is *dorsiflexion* of the ankle and inversion (turning the sole

inwards) of the foot. (See the diagram on page 202.)

Till – *til* – a drawer or tray that contains money.

Time management – *t-eye-m man-aj-men-t* – the process of planning, organising and controlling activities that will allow the most effective use of time.

Tinea pedis – *tin-ee-a ped-is* – see *athlete's foot*.

Tint – *tin-t* – a commercial dye used to change the colour of eyelashes and brows. *Also* a shade of colour.

Tissue – *ti-sh-you* – a group of *cells*, fibres and various cell products that form a structure or substance and perform a similar function. There are four types of tissue in the body: *epithelial tissue*, *connective tissue*, *muscle* and *nerves*.

Tissue fluid – *ti-sh-you fl-oo-id* – a watery solution that leaks out of *capillaries* and surrounds and bathes the cells. Also known as *interstitial fluid* or *intercellular fluid*.

173

Tocopherol – *tok-of-er-ol* – the technical term for vitamin E, a fat-soluble (capable of being dissolved in fat) *vitamin*. It is an important **antioxidant**. It has healing properties and helps to repair sun-damaged skin. It is found in nuts, seeds, leafy green vegetables and vegetable oils.

Toe nail clippers – *t-oh-nay-l k-lip-per-s* – a metal implement used to cut and shorten the toe nails.

Toe separator – *t-oh sep-a-ray-t-or* – a disposable implement placed between the toes to separate them and allow enamelling of the toe nails without smudging.

Tone – *t-oh-n* – to tighten and firm, to strengthen. *Also* the normal state of elastic tension or partial **contraction** in resting muscles. *Also* a quality of colour. *Also* a distinctive sound or pitch of the voice.

Toning lotion – *t-oh-n-in-g lo-sh-on* – a product applied to the skin after cleansing to remove excess grease, tighten the pores and refresh the skin. It may also be used as an active ingredient in a clay **face mask**, mixed with a special powder.

Top coat – *top-k-oh-t* – the final coat of enamel applied over the base coat and colour to protect and provide a glossy finish to a **manicure** or **pedicure**.

Toxic – *tok-sik* – poisonous, having the effect of a poison.

Toxin – *tok-sin* – a poison, any substance that has a toxic effect on the body.

Trading Standards Service – *t-ray-din-g st-an-d-ar-d-s ser-vis* – a government department the role of which is to promote and maintain fair trading, protect consumers and enable reputable businesses to thrive. It enforces a wide range of consumer **legislation** (laws) in order to protect consumers and honest businesses. It also provides advice to businesses in order to help them comply with the law.

Training – *tr-ay-nin-g* –
education and instruction to
teach a new skill or increase
knowledge.

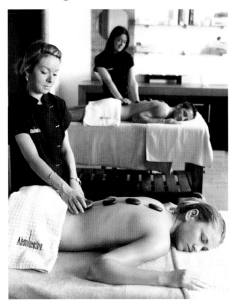

A training session in hot stone massage

Transfers – *t-ran-s-fer-s* – a
form of instant nail art, including
flat and three-dimensional nail
designs. Transfers are available as
self-adhesive designs, which are
peeled off the backing sheet and
applied to the nail, or as water-
release 'decals' (transfers) which
may be removed from the backing
sheet when it is wet and then
applied to the enamelled nail
before applying a top coat.

Transformer – *tr-an-s-for-mer*
– an electrical device that reduces
the voltage (strength – see **volt**)
of an **alternating current**.

Transparent layer – *tr-ans-p-a-
r-ent lay-er* – see **stratum
lucidum**.

Transversus abdominis –
tranz-ver-sus ab-dom-in-is – the
deep **muscle** of the lower
abdomen, extending from the
iliac crest (hip bone) and lower six
ribs to the linea alba (fibrous
tissue in a band down the centre
of the abdominal wall) and pubis
(a bone in the **pelvic girdle**). Its
action is to compress (squeeze)
the abdomen.

Trapezius – *tr-ap-ee-z-ee-us* –
a broad, flat **muscle** on each side
of the upper back, shoulders and
neck. It raises, rotates and draws
back the shoulders and pulls the
head backward or to one side.

Traveller's cheque – *tr-av-e-
ler-s ch-ek* – a form of **currency**
used mainly when travelling to
another country. The cheque must
be signed when purchased and it
may be offered as payment for
goods. It requires presentation of
the holder's passport and *(continued)*

it must be signed again in the presence of the vendor so that the signature may be verified against the original.

Treat – tr-ee-t – to provide a *therapy* in order to meet objectives.

Treatment – t-ree-t-men-t – the carrying out or application of a facial or body *therapy* in order to help remedy a problem or make an improvement.

Treatment advice – t-ree-t-men-t ad-v-eye-s – recommendations offered as a guide when deciding on the correct *therapies* to meet the client's objectives.

Treatment plan – tr-ee-t-men-t pl-an – a record to show the *treatment* programme required to achieve agreed objectives. This will include skin, body or nail *analysis*, suggested treatments, frequency of treatments, home care products and *lifestyle* advice.

Triceps – tr-eye-sep-s – the *muscle* on the back of the upper arm. It extends (straightens) the forearm. (See the diagram on page 202.)

Trigeminal nerve – tr-eye-jem-in-al n-er-v – the fifth facial *nerve*. It is the largest cranial (located in the *cranium*) nerve and has three branches: ophthalmic, maxillary and mandibular. It consists of: motor (producing movement) fibres that activate the muscles of mastication (chewing); and sensory (receiving messages) fibres that carry impulses (signals) from the head and face to the brain.

Tri-iodothyronine – tr-eye-eye-oh-doh-th-eye-roh-n-eye-n – a *hormone* produced by the *thyroid gland* that increases the *metabolic rate* and regulates *protein*, fat and *carbohydrate metabolism*.

Tumour – t-you-mor – a swelling or enlargement, a group of abnormal cells. Tumours may be *benign* (harmless) or *malignant* (cancerous).

Turban – ter-ban – a towelling head covering to protect the client's hair during facial treatment.

Turnover – *ter-n-oh-ver* – the amount of money received by a business in a given period.

Tweezers – *t-wee-zer-s* – small metal pincers used to pluck hairs or to pick up small objects.

Tyrosinase – *t-eye-roh-sin-ay-s* – an *enzyme* that stimulates *melanin* production.

Tyrosine – *t-eye-roh-see-n* – an *amino acid* that initiates the production of *melanin* in the skin.

Ulna – *ul-na* – the bone of the forearm on the side opposite to the thumb. (See the diagram on page 197.)

Ultrasound – *ul-t-ra-sow-n-d* – sound waves of a very high *frequency* (above 20,000 *Hertz*).

Ultraviolet (UV) radiation – *ul-t-ra-v-eye-oh-let r-ay-s* – invisible short-wavelength *radiation* beyond the violet end of the visible light spectrum. UVA rays have a *wavelength* of 320–400 nanometres (320–400 thousand-millionths of a metre) and cause changes in the skin such as *inflammation*, abnormal cell production, thickening of the *stratum corneum*, reduction in the number of cells that stimulate the immune response and *elastin* deterioration (worsening of quality). UVB rays have a wavelength of 290–320 nanometres and cause sunburn. Also known as ultraviolet rays or UV rays.

Unsafe behaviour – *un-say-f bee-hay-v-yor* – action that may cause harm to self or others.

Urea – *you-ree-a* – a product of protein *metabolism*. It is produced commercially from synthetic ammonia and *carbon dioxide* and used in face creams, hair conditioners and body lotions.

Urinary system – *you-r-eye-n-a-ree sis-t-em* – the body system that provides a filtering mechanism for the blood, regulates water and salt levels in the body and excretes (removes from the body) waste. It maintains the volume (amount) and composition of body fluids within normal limits. It includes the kidneys, bladder, ureters and urethra.

Urine – *you-r-in* – the liquid waste matter excreted (removed from the body) by the kidneys.

Urticaria – *er-tik-air-ee-a* – see *hives*.

Uterus – *you-ter-us* – the womb.

UV tanning – *you-vee tan-in-g* – the production of a tan in response to exposure to *ultraviolet radiation*, either naturally from the sun or artificially from sun beds and other tanning equipment. UV radiation is divided into A and B rays. UVA rays penetrate into the *dermis*, providing an immediate but temporary colour. They generate *free radicals* that alter the skin cells and fibres and contribute to the ageing of the skin. UVB rays penetrate into the *epidermis*, stimulating the production of vitamin D, which is needed for growth and healthy bones. UVB rays are, however, responsible for burning the skin and in some cases contribute to the formation of skin cancer.

Vacuum – *vak-you-m* – an empty space containing no matter. Also an enclosed space where the air has been partially removed so the air remaining in the space exerts less pressure than the surrounding atmosphere.

Vacuum suction – *vak-you-m suk-shon* – a mechanical method of *lymph drainage* used to stimulate the *lymphatic system* and so speed up the removal of waste from the body and disperse (get rid of) fluid from the *tissues*. It is applied using a vacuum suction unit containing an electrically driven vacuum pump connected to a perspex or glass *ventouse* (cup) by a flexible plastic tube. The pump draws air from the ventouse causing the air pressure inside to drop. This forms a partial *vacuum* that lifts the underlying *tissue* up into the ventouse, which is then slowly guided over the skin towards the *lymph nodes*.

Valve – *val-v* – a membranous (made of *membrane*) structure in a hollow organ, passage or vessel that folds or closes to prevent backflow of fluid. Also a device that controls the flow of gases, liquids or other materials through a passage.

Variable cost – *vair-ee-ab-l kos-t* – a cost that varies depending on the treatment provided.

Varicose vein – *var-ik-oh-s v-ay-n* – a distended (stretched) **vein** occurring most commonly in the legs. The condition is often inherited or caused by obstruction to blood flow. Extra care must be taken during *treatment*. Some treatments may be contraindicated (see *contraindication*) or treatment may need to be adapted or modified.

Varnish – *var-ni-sh* – the coating of a surface used to add colour and gloss. *Also* another name for enamel.

Vasoconstriction – *vay-so-kon-st-rik-sh-on* – decrease in diameter of *blood vessels*.

Vasodilation – *vay-so-d-eye-lay-shon* – increase in diameter of *blood vessels*.

Vasopressin – *vay-so-pre-sin* – see *antidiuretic hormone*.

VAT – *vee-ay-tee* – stands for value **added tax**: a tax on consumer spending on goods and services. A business must register for VAT when its taxable *turnover* reaches a certain limit.

Vein – *v-ay-n* – a *blood vessel* that carries blood towards the heart.

Vellus hair – *vel-us h-air* – the fine, soft, downy hair of the foetus (unborn baby) that covers some parts of the body.

Venous return – *vee-n-us re-ter-n* – the flow of blood back to the heart.

Ventouse – *von-too-s* – a glass or perspex cup used in *vacuum suction*.

Ventricle – *ven-tr-ik-l* – either of the two lower chambers (right and left) of the heart that collect blood from the *atria*, the smaller chambers above, and pump it out of the heart. (See the diagram on page 198.) Also part of the body filled with fluid.

Venule – *ven-you-l* – a minute *blood vessel* that drains blood from the *capillaries* and carries it towards the *veins*.

Verruca plantaris – *ve-roo-k-a pl-an-tar-is* – a *wart* occurring on the sole of the foot. Also known as plantar wart.

Vertebra – *ver-te-br-a* (plural **vertebrae** – *ver-te-br-ay*) – the vertebrae are the bones of the spinal column. Each vertebra contains an arched hollow section through which the spinal cord (part of the *central nervous system*) passes and is separated from its neighbour by a disc. The spinal column is divided into sections of vertebrae: 7 cervical (in the neck), 12 thoracic (in the chest and rib cage), 5 lumbar (in the lower back), 5 sacral (in the pelvis) and 4 that form the coccyx. Some sacral bones and some bones of the coccyx fuse together in adulthood. (See the diagram on page 196.)

Vesicle – *ves-ik-l* – a tiny *blister* in the skin containing a clear fluid.

Vibrations – *v-eye-br-ay-shon-s* – fine, trembling *massage* manipulations that are gentle and soothing in effect, using the palmar (front) surface of the hands and the fingertips on the area to be treated. The vibrations are achieved by rapid *(continued)*

contraction and relaxation of the muscles in the therapist's arms and hands.

Vichy shower – vi-sh-ee sh-ow-er – a popular spa **treatment** in which the client lies on a wet table and a fine spray of water is produced by microjets fixed to a horizontal rail above the table. The temperature of the water and the pressure of the spray may be altered to suit each individual client and the therapist can apply massage to the body at the same time. The effects are soothing or stimulating depending on the pressure of the water jets. Also known as an affusion shower.

Virilism – vi-ril-is-m – the development of masculine characteristics in a female – e.g. deepening of the voice and increased body hair and muscle bulk.

Virus – v-eye-rus – a micro-organism (a tiny organism that can't be seen with the naked eye) that causes disease. Viruses are smaller than **bacteria** and

capable of reproduction and mutation (sudden **genetic** change) in living cells.

Vitamins – vit-a-min-s – essential substances required in small amounts for healthy growth and development in the body.

Vitiligo – vit-i-l-eye-go – the gradual appearance of single or multiple white areas of skin on any part of the body due to the destruction of **melanocytes**. The skin sometimes becomes totally devoid of **pigment**. The areas of white skin are prone to burning in the sun and must be well protected. Also known as leucoderma.

Volt – v-o-l-t – a unit of electricity measuring the force driving electricity through a circuit.

Voluntary – vol-un-ta-ree – done willingly without being forced or obliged to do it.

Voluntary muscle – vol-un-ta-ree mu-sel – see **skeletal muscle**.

Warm wax – *w-or-m wa-ks* – a depilatory (removes hair) wax with a low melting point of 43°C used to remove *superfluous* hair from the body. It may be made from paraffin wax mixed with other substances such as rubber latex solution, *solvents* or organic honey. It is applied thinly with a spatula in the direction of hair growth and removed with a muslin or paper strip against the hair growth. Some warm waxes are used cold in the form of strips impregnated (soaked) with wax and are available for use by the client at home.

Wart – *w-or-t* – a *benign* (harmless) growth on the skin caused by a *virus*, specifically the human papillomavirus (HPV). Warts are areas of skin that grow faster than normal, are skin-coloured, feel rough to the touch and are most common on the hands, feet and face. There are several types of wart: verruca vulgaris or common wart (mostly found on hands and knees); verruca plana (a flat, tan or flesh-coloured wart, sometimes occurring in large numbers on the face, neck, hands, wrists and knees); verruca filiform (a thread-like wart most common on the face and neck); *verruca plantaris* or plantar wart (found on pressure points on the soles of the feet).

Waste material – *w-ay-s-t mat-ee-r-ee-al* – used and unwanted products or by-products from performing face and body *treatments* or from other procedures such as *sanitising*, which must be disposed of safely and hygienically. Normal waste should be placed in a plastic-lined bin with a lid; broken glass and used needles and other sharp objects must be placed in a *Sharps box*; and contaminated waste must be placed in a yellow plastic-lined bin for removal by a licensed waste disposal company.

Water testing kit – *w-or-ter tes-tin-g kit* – a set of equipment used to test the cleanliness of the water in a spa or swimming pool, helping to promote a healthy and safe environment for bathers. It allows the operator to test for free and combined chlorine and the alkalinity (level of *alkaline*) of the water.

Watery eyes – *w-or-t-er-ee eye-s* – an overflow of tears due to excessive *secretion* (continued) from the lacrimal (tear) **glands**. Also known as epiphora.

Watt – *wot* – a unit of electrical power.

Wavelength – *w-ay-v-len-g-th* – the distance between repeating units of a wave pattern that transfers energy from one point to another, e.g. electromagnetic waves (see **electromagnetic spectrum**) and **electric current**.

Wax – *w-aks* – traditionally a substance secreted (produced) by bees called beeswax. Now different types of wax exist, both natural and synthetic. Two forms of wax with properties similar to beeswax are paraffin (a petroleum wax) and carnauba (a vegetable wax). They both have a melting point above 45°C, form a liquid when melted, are malleable (easy to shape) at room temperature, insoluble (cannot be dissolved) in water and hydrophobic (repel water). Wax is used to make candles, in **depilation**, in makeup and in **face masks**.

Wax heater – *w-aks hee-t-er* – a thermostatically (see **thermostat**) controlled container

for depilatory wax (wax used in **depilation**).

Waxing strip – *w-aks-in-g st-rip-s* – a narrow piece of muslin or paper used to remove **warm wax** that has been applied to the skin to remove **superfluous** hair.

Weakness – *wee-k-nes-es* – a defect or failing.

White blood cell – *w-eye-t bl-ud sel-s* – an important part of the **immune system**, white blood cells are a component of blood and are produced in the bone marrow (soft tissue in the centre of bones). They help to defend the body against disease. These **cells** are also found in large numbers in the spleen and **lymphatic system**. There are two different categories: granulocytes and agranulocytes. Granulocytes include: neutrophils (which respond quickly to bacterial **infection**); basophils (which release the chemical **histamine** in response to **allergy**); and eosinophils (which deal mainly with **parasitic infections**). There are two types of agranulocytes: monocytes (which are responsible for engulfing and digesting **bacteria** and foreign substances in the blood – monocytes that migrate from (move out of) blood are called *macrophages*); and *lymphocytes* (which make *antibodies*, coordinate the immune response and destroy infected cells). Also known as leucocyte.

White skin – *w-eye-t sk-in* – this skin produces smaller amounts of *melanin* than darker skin. In some cases it is very pale with *freckles* and can be accompanied by blonde or red hair and blue or green eyes. There is a higher risk of sunburn and the formation of skin cancer because of the reduced protection from lack of melanin in the skin. Some white skins tan more easily and are less sensitive, such as Scandinavian skins, which, although pale, develop a tan in the summer months without burning. In general, white skin ages faster than *black skin*, and requires more protection from the environment and the sun's rays.

Whitehead – *w-eye-t-hed* – see *milium*.

Whitlow – *wit-l-oh* – see *paronychia*.

Witch hazel – *wit-ch hay-z-el* – an *astringent* used to tighten the *pores*, cool the skin, remove surface oil and cosmetic preparations and as an ingredient in a *face mask*.

Wood's light – *w-ud-s l-eye-t* – a lamp emitting long-wave ultraviolet radiation (UVA rays) used to examine the skin.

Working capital – *wer-kin-g kap-it-al* – the money that is readily available for day-to-day business expenses – the difference between *current assets* and current liabilities (money that the business has to spend within one year).

Working practices – *wer-kin-g pr-ak-tis-es* – the agreed method of performing *treatments*, tasks and other *duties* when carrying out a particular job.

Working temperature – *wer-kin-g tem-pe-rat-your* – the optimum (ideal) temperature at which a thermostatically controlled piece of equipment works most effectively. Also the ideal temperature in which to work. Health and safety regulations set the *(continued)* minimum legal working temperature at 13–16°C. There is no maximum working temperature but the approved code of practice states that 'all reasonable steps should be taken to achieve a comfortable working temperature'. Reasonable steps might include providing suitable fans or air conditioning.

Workplace policy – *wer-k-pl-ay-s pol-i-see* – a statement to guide decisions and actions and form the basis of workplace rules. A salon owner will state their policy regarding *health and safety*, using *hazardous substances*, emergency procedures, personal presentation and smoking, eating and drinking in the salon. They will provide their employees with a list of rules to help them follow the company policies. Policies in other areas may be also be stated, such as dealing with returns and refunds, customer complaints, employee lateness and absence and *confidentiality*.

Wrap – *r-ap* – a thin coating applied to the natural nail or an application over a plastic nail tip. Strengthening wraps are made from silk or fibreglass. Also known as an overlay. See also *body wrap*.

Wringing – *rin-g-in-g* – a *massage* manipulation which involves compressing tissue between the thumbs and index fingers and then pulling it from side to side, working along the length of the *muscle*. It increases circulation, warms the skin and relaxes the client.

Wrinkles – *rin-k-l-s* – fine surface lines or deep furrows in the skin that appear on sun-exposed areas of the body and increase with age. The main causes are related to ageing, as *collagen* and *elastin* break down and the moisture levels in the skin decrease, also habitual facial expressions, gravity and damage from the environment and *ultraviolet radiation*.

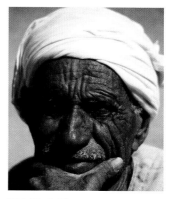

Wrinkled skin

Wrist extensors – *ris-t x-ten-s-or-s* – the **muscles** on the **posterior** aspect (back) of the lower arm that bend the wrist **joint** backwards, moving the back of the hand toward the back of the forearm. (See the diagram on page 202.)

Wrist flexors – *ris-t fl-ex-or-s* – the muscles on the **anterior** aspect (front) of the lower arm that bend the wrist **joint** forwards, moving the palm of the hand toward the front of the forearm. (See the diagram on page 202.)

Xanthoma – *zan-th-oh-ma* – a yellow-coloured skin **lesion** which is associated with disorders of fat **metabolism** and high levels of **cholesterol** in the blood.

Zinc – *zin-k* – a trace (found in small amounts) element with anti-irritant and **antioxidant** effects.

Zygomatic bone – *z-eye-go-mat-ik b-oh-n* – the cheek bone. (See the diagram on page 196.)

Zygomaticus major – *z-eye-go-mat-ik-us may-jor* – a band of **muscle** on each side of the face, from the **zygomatic bone** to the muscle around the mouth. It pulls the corner of the mouth upward and backward as in laughing or smiling broadly. (See the diagram on page 192.)

Zygomaticus minor – *z-eye-go-mat-ik-us m-eye-n-or* – smaller than the **zygomaticus major**, this **muscle** is situated on either side of the face, from the **zygomatic bone** to the upper lip. It raises the upper lip as in smiling. (See the diagram on page 192.)

Appendix

The structure of a cell

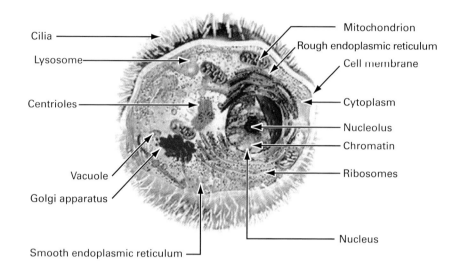

Cilia

Lysosome

Centrioles

Vacuole

Golgi apparatus

Smooth endoplasmic reticulum

Mitochondrion

Rough endoplasmic reticulum

Cell membrane

Cytoplasm

Nucleolus

Chromatin

Ribosomes

Nucleus

Cell membrane is a thin flexible barrier around cells of organisms; it controls the chemicals entering and leaving the cell

Centrioles participate in the early stages of cell division

Chromatin threads which carry DNA

Cilia tiny, thin hair like projections extending from some cell membranes for movement of the cell or the surrounding medium

Cytoplasm contains nutrients necessary for growth, reproduction and repair

Endoplasmic reticulum is a network within cytoplasm involved in the synthesis, modification and transportation of cellular material

Golgi apparatus an organelle responsible for the modification and transport of proteins

Lysosomes are organelles containing enzymes

Mitochondrion provides the energy for cellular activity

Nucleolus manufactures ribosomes

Nucleus is the control centre of the cell

Ribosomes make proteins for the cell

Vacuole stores and releases cellular waste products

The structure of the skin

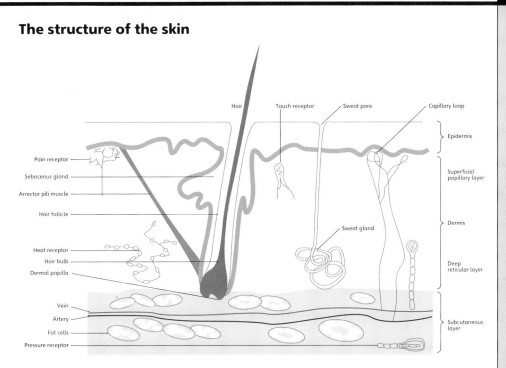

Hair | Touch receptor | Sweat pore | Capillary loop

Epidermis

Pain receptor
Sebaceous gland
Arrector pili muscle
Hair follicle

Superficial papillary layer

Sweat gland

Dermis

Heat receptor
Hair bulb
Dermal papilla

Deep reticular layer

Vein
Artery
Fat cells
Pressure receptor

Subcutaneous layer

The structure of the epidermis

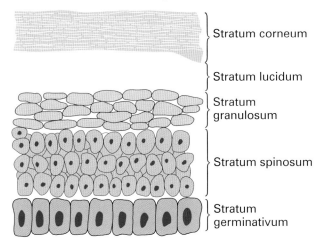

Stratum corneum

Stratum lucidum

Stratum granulosum

Stratum spinosum

Stratum germinativum

Appendix

The structure of the nail

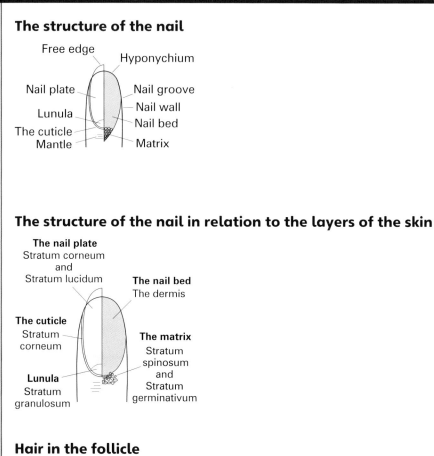

Free edge
Hyponychium
Nail plate
Nail groove
Lunula
Nail wall
Nail bed
The cuticle
Mantle
Matrix

The structure of the nail in relation to the layers of the skin

The nail plate
Stratum corneum
and
Stratum lucidum

The nail bed
The dermis

The cuticle
Stratum
corneum

The matrix
Stratum
spinosum
and
Stratum
germinativum

Lunula
Stratum
granulosum

Hair in the follicle

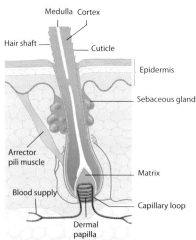

Medulla Cortex
Hair shaft
Cuticle
Epidermis
Sebaceous gland
Arrector
pili muscle
Blood supply
Matrix
Capillary loop
Dermal
papilla

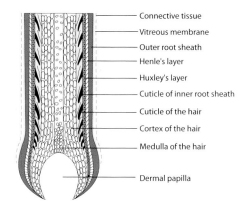

Connective tissue
Vitreous membrane
Outer root sheath
Henle's layer
Huxley's layer
Cuticle of inner root sheath
Cuticle of the hair
Cortex of the hair
Medulla of the hair
Dermal papilla

Cross-section of the hair and follicle

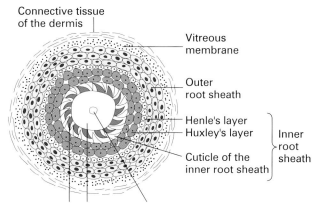

Connective tissue of the dermis

Vitreous membrane

Outer root sheath

Henle's layer
Huxley's layer
Cuticle of the inner root sheath

Inner root sheath

Hair cuticle   Hair cortex   Hair medulla

Cross-section of the hair

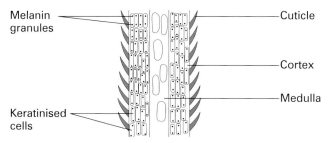

Melanin granules

Cuticle

Cortex

Medulla

Keratinised cells

The hair growth cycle and stages of follicle development

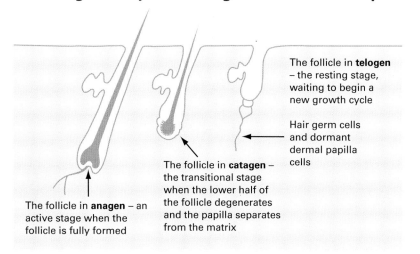

The follicle in **telogen** – the resting stage, waiting to begin a new growth cycle

Hair germ cells and dormant dermal papilla cells

The follicle in **catagen** – the transitional stage when the lower half of the follicle degenerates and the papilla separates from the matrix

The follicle in **anagen** – an active stage when the follicle is fully formed

The muscles of the face and neck

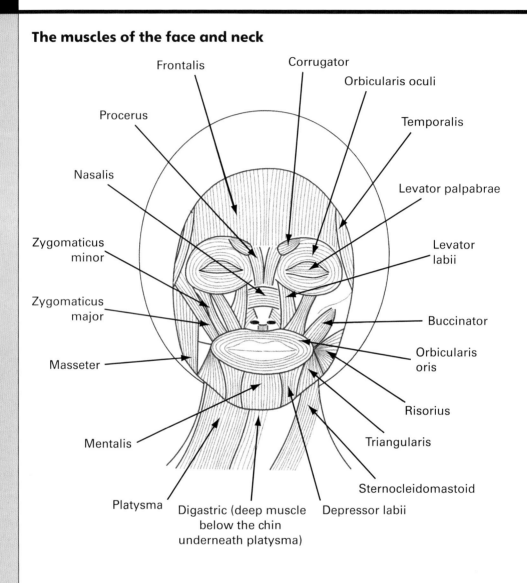

Frontalis

Corrugator

Orbicularis oculi

Temporalis

Procerus

Levator palpabrae

Nasalis

Levator labii

Zygomaticus minor

Zygomaticus major

Buccinator

Masseter

Orbicularis oris

Risorius

Mentalis

Triangularis

Sternocleidomastoid

Platysma

Digastric (deep muscle below the chin underneath platysma)

Depressor labii

Position and action of the superficial muscles of the face and neck

Muscle	Position	Action
Occipitalis	Covers the occipital bone, back of the scalp	Draws the scalp backwards
Frontalis	Covers the frontal bone, front of the scalp and over the forehead	Draws the scalp forwards, raises the eyebrows and wrinkles the forehead horizontally
Corrugator	The inside corner of each eyebrow	Draws the eyebrows together causing vertical furrows
Procerus	The top of the nose between the eyes	Depresses the eyebrow and causes wrinkles across the bridge of the nose
Orbicularis oculi	Around the eye	Closes the eyes tightly
Levator palpabrae	The eyelid	Opens the upper lid
Nasalis	Immediately below the procerus, across the bridge of the nose	Compresses the nasal openings
Levator labii	From the outer edge of the mouth up and over the maxilla	Raises the upper lip
Zygomaticus – major and minor	The skin and fascia at the angle of the mouth to the zygomatic bone	Raises the lips as in laughing
Risorius	From the corner of the mouth across the cheek	Draws the corners of the mouth out and back as in grinning

Muscle	Position	Action
Buccinator	From the corner of the mouth, outwards and upwards across the cheek	Compresses the cheeks and aids in mastication
Orbicularis oris	Around the mouth	Closes the mouth and causes the lips to wrinkle. Also puckers the lips as in kissing
Triangularis	From the corner of the lower lip to the chin	Pulls the corner of the mouth down
Depressor labii	From the mandible to the lower lip	Pulls the lower lip down and to one side
Mentalis	Over the chin	Pushes up the lower lip, wrinkling the chin
Temporalis	From the temple down to the jaw	Raises the lower jaw and draws it backwards. Helps with chewing
Masseter	From the cheekbone down to the angle of the jaw	Raises the jaw. Helps with chewing
Platysma	Covers the front of the neck	Helps draw down the mandible and lower lip and wrinkles the skin of the neck
Sternocleido-mastoid	The side of the neck from the ear to the clavicle and the sternum	Both sides together flex the neck. One side alone bends the head sideways
Digastric	The deep muscle under the chin attached to the mandible, temporal and hyoid bones	Helps in moving the tongue and swallowing

Charts with names and number of bones

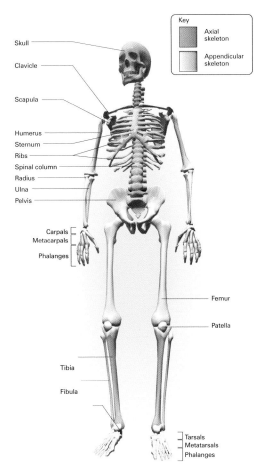

Skull		
Clavicle		
Scapula		
Humerus		
Sternum		
Ribs		
Spinal column		
Radius		
Ulna		
Pelvis		
Carpals		
Metacarpals		
Phalanges		
		Femur
		Patella
Tibia		
Fibula		
		Tarsals
		Metatarsals
		Phalanges

Key
Axial skeleton
Appendicular skeleton

Axial skeleton			
1 frontal	4 nasal	7 cervical vertebrae	
2 parietal	1 vomer	12 thoracic vertebrae	
2 temporal	1 maxilla	5 lumbar vertebrae	
1 occipital	1 mandible	5 fused bones of sacrum	
1 ethmoid	2 zygomatic	4 fused bones of coccyx	
1 sphenoid	2 palatine	24 (12 pairs) ribs	
2 lacrimal	1 hyoid	1 sternum	**Total 80 bones**

Appendix

The vertebral column

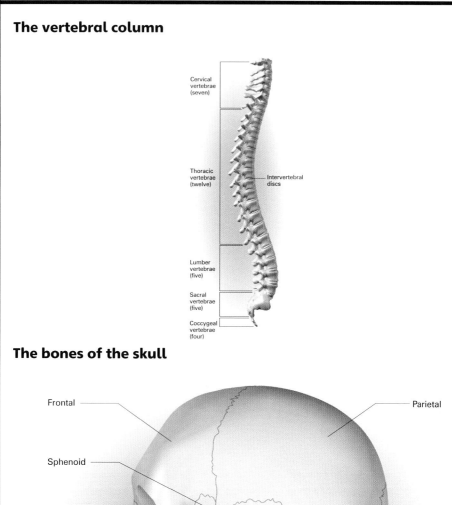

Cervical vertebrae (seven)

Thoracic vertebrae (twelve)

Intervertebral discs

Lumber vertebrae (five)

Sacral vertebrae (five)

Coccygeal vertebrae (four)

The bones of the skull

Frontal

Parietal

Sphenoid

Nasal

Ethmoid

Zygomatic

Occipital

Maxilla

Temporal

Mandible

The bones of the hand, wrist and forearm

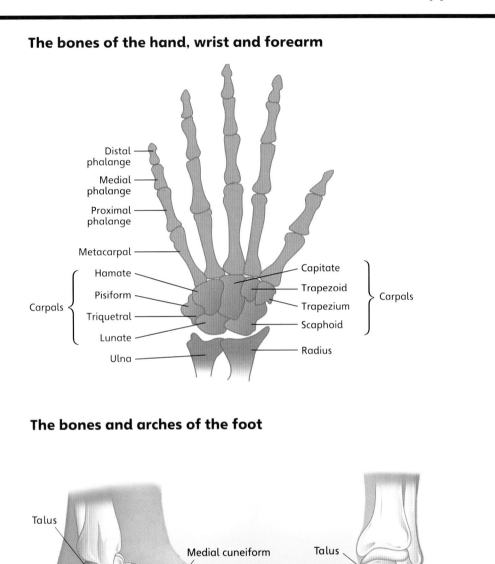

Distal phalange
Medial phalange
Proximal phalange
Metacarpal
Carpals
Hamate
Pisiform
Triquetral
Lunate
Ulna
Capitate
Trapezoid
Trapezium
Scaphoid
Carpals
Radius

The bones and arches of the foot

Talus
Medial cuneiform
Metatarsals
Talus
Metatarsals
Transverse arch
Calcaneus
Lateral longitudinal arch
Medial longitudinal arch

Appendix

The heart

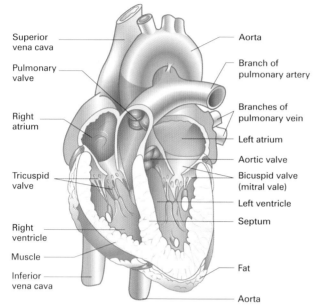

- Superior vena cava
- Pulmonary valve
- Right atrium
- Tricuspid valve
- Right ventricle
- Muscle
- Inferior vena cava

- Aorta
- Branch of pulmonary artery
- Branches of pulmonary vein
- Left atrium
- Aortic valve
- Bicuspid valve (mitral vale)
- Left ventricle
- Septum
- Fat
- Aorta

The path of blood through the heart

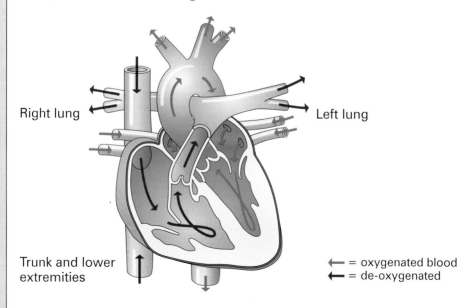

Right lung

Left lung

Trunk and lower extremities

⟵ = oxygenated blood
⬅ = de-oxygenated

The pulmonary and systemic circulatory systems

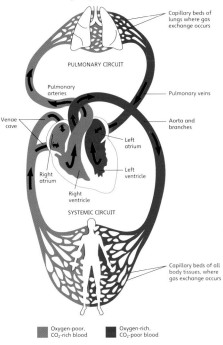

The lymphatic system and the lymph organs

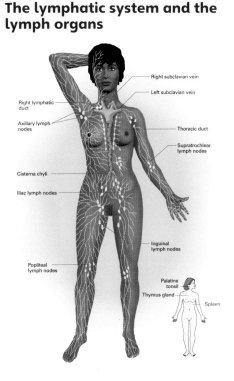

The lymph nodes of the face and neck

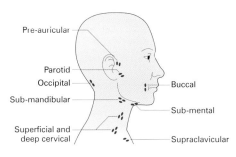

A cross-section of a lymph node

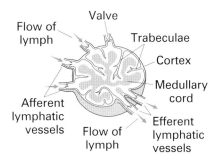

Appendix

The endocrine glands

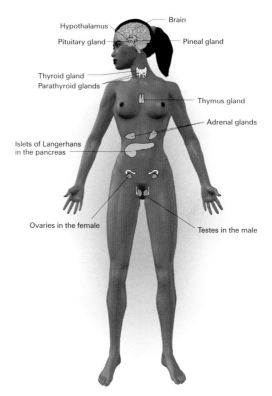

The hormones secreted by the pituitary gland

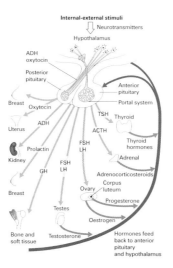

The spinal nerves

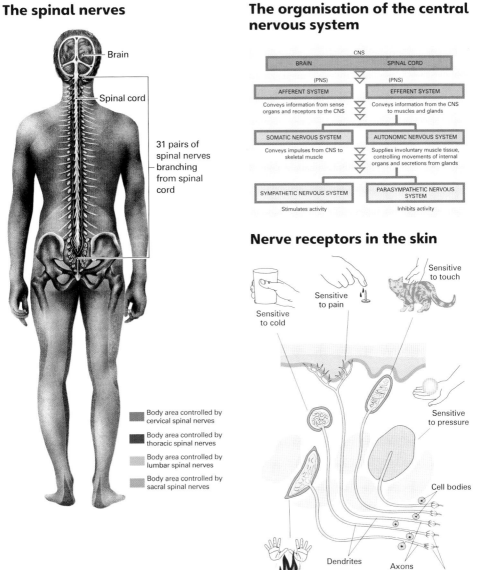

Brain

Spinal cord

31 pairs of spinal nerves branching from spinal cord

Body area controlled by cervical spinal nerves

Body area controlled by thoracic spinal nerves

Body area controlled by lumbar spinal nerves

Body area controlled by sacral spinal nerves

The organisation of the central nervous system

CNS

BRAIN	SPINAL CORD

(PNS)   (PNS)

AFFERENT SYSTEM	EFFERENT SYSTEM
Conveys information from sense organs and receptors to the CNS	Conveys information from the CNS to muscles and glands

SOMATIC NERVOUS SYSTEM	AUTONOMIC NERVOUS SYSTEM
Conveys impulses from CNS to skeletal muscle	Supplies involuntary muscle tissue, controlling movements of internal organs and secretions from glands

SYMPATHETIC NERVOUS SYSTEM	PARASYMPATHETIC NERVOUS SYSTEM
Stimulates activity	Inhibits activity

Nerve receptors in the skin

Sensitive to cold

Sensitive to pain

Sensitive to touch

Sensitive to pressure

Cell bodies

Dendrites

Axons

Synapses

Sensitive to heat

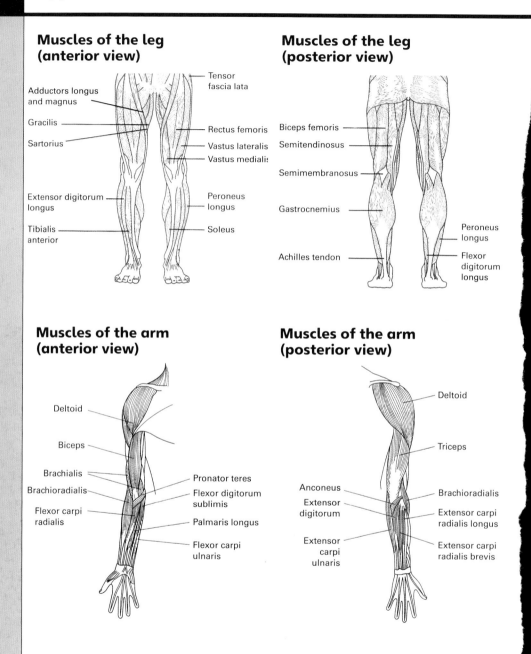

Muscles of the leg (anterior view)

Adductors longus and magnus
Gracilis
Sartorius
Tensor fascia lata
Rectus femoris
Vastus lateralis
Vastus medialis
Extensor digitorum longus
Tibialis anterior
Peroneus longus
Soleus

Muscles of the leg (posterior view)

Biceps femoris
Semitendinosus
Semimembranosus
Gastrocnemius
Achilles tendon
Peroneus longus
Flexor digitorum longus

Muscles of the arm (anterior view)

Deltoid
Biceps
Brachialis
Brachioradialis
Flexor carpi radialis
Pronator teres
Flexor digitorum sublimis
Palmaris longus
Flexor carpi ulnaris

Muscles of the arm (posterior view)

Deltoid
Triceps
Anconeus
Extensor digitorum
Extensor carpi ulnaris
Brachioradialis
Extensor carpi radialis longus
Extensor carpi radialis brevis